Mary Ellen Pinkham lives in Minneapolis with her husband and son. Her three previous bestsellers on kitchen and household hints have sold over seven million copies and she is now one of America's most successful and sought-after personalities.

Mary Ellen Pinkham

Mary Ellen's Help Yourself Diet Plan*

*The One That Worked For Me

Fontana Paperbacks

First published in the USA
by St Martin's Press/Marek 1983
First published in Great Britain
by Fontana Paperbacks 1983

Copyright © Mary Ellen Pinkham
and Dale Ronda Burg 1983

Set in 10 on 11 pt Linotron Plantin

Made and printed in Great Britain by
William Collins Sons & Co. Ltd, Glasgow

A hardback edition is published by
William Collins Sons & Co. Ltd

Grateful acknowledgment is made for
permission to abridge the listing on page 206,
from pages 154–5 in *Food Values of Portions
Commonly Used* (thirteenth edition) by Jean
A. T. Pennington and Helen Nichols Church.
Copyright © 1980 by Helen Nichols Church,
BS, and Jean A. T. Pennington, PhD, RD.
Reprinted by permission of Harper & Row
Publishers, Inc.

Grateful acknowledgment is also made to
Maggie Black, who converted the American
ingredients and measures for the UK edition.

This book is dedicated to Sherman F. Pinkham, Jr, the man I live with, and Jonathan Lazear, the man I work with.

Contents

Part Three Second Helpings

Acknowledgments

I'd like to acknowledge the help of lots and lots of people, but I've been told I've only got room here for a few. I'd like to single out for thanks:

Dale Burg, my collaborator and sounding board, whose help and support saw me through this project. She's the best!

Dr Joel Holger, my internist, a wonderful find: a man who knows his ABCs – and a few other important letters – in the nutrition field. I want to thank him for his guidance and patience.

Judith C. Goldberg, nutritionist extraordinaire, whose doctoral work was in the area of obesity. Judy helped me out in every phase of this project. She's some smart cookie!

C. B. Abbott, whose research was great. When several nutritionists saw the material Connie dug up, they were amazed. The CIA would be lucky to have a researcher like her.

Walter C. Hewett, an ex-chronic dieter, now a weight counsellor. Walter finally came to grips with everything that chronic dieting entails and wound up a good (and thin) adviser and example.

Samuel Kaplan, my lawyer. He's my friend, too. Everyone on earth should have that combo, but not everyone is as lucky as I am. He supported me all the way.

Tom Oberg, George Cleveland, Kathy Rice, and Wendy Lazear, members of the Mary Ellen Enterprises staff. Behind the scenes, they helped in many ways and were always there for me.

Andrew Pinkham, my son. When he told his Mum she reminded him of the little fat mouse in *Cinderella*, he sure started something . . .

Foreword

I've already offered my congratulations to Mary Ellen Pinkham – the new Mary Ellen Pinkham, nearly eighty pounds leaner and more fit than when I first met her. Now I congratulate you for starting this book. I am sure you'll find it a treat to read, and I think it contains more than a few surprises. This book can change your life, if you let it.

When Mary Ellen came to us, she was complaining of flu: she was tired, worn out, and feverish. But even before she'd become ill, she hadn't felt well. She was significantly overweight and tired of constant dieting without much result.

She told me that she'd been on one diet or another for as long as she could remember – all failures. She didn't realize, until I told her, that that was the key to her problem. She was a victim of dieting. Fad dieting had changed her metabolism so that she could never hope to lose weight and keep it off.

My practice is not oriented towards the treatment of obesity, but as an internist I estimate that nearly half of my patients are concerned about being too overweight. Rarely does a day go by without a patient asking my advice about diets or dieting. And, often, the stories I hear are similar to Mary Ellen's. The patient has lost weight on diet after diet, then regained it all and often a few extra pounds.

It seemed to me that there were certain basic, scientific principles that most dieters were failing to take into account. It further seemed possible to devise a programme that incorporated these principles.

When I got to know Mary Ellen a little better and we discussed the extent of her problem, she was very excited by the information I shared with her. She said she felt that was the first time she really got the truth about diets and dieting.

What I explained to her was not difficult to understand, but it was up to her to put the ideas into effect once we'd worked out a plan, for we agreed she would be the subject to provide the findings of current research. Together, we found ways to help Mary Ellen change her metabolism and get rid of inappropriate eating habits. As soon as she began to get results, Mary Ellen made the commitment to follow through and the ultimate promise to herself that she would adhere to this new way of living on a life-long basis.

What follows is the story of Mary Ellen's experience and the plan that worked for her. You'll enjoy it, because everyone likes to read a success story. What you should especially enjoy is the knowledge that her success can be duplicated by others. The plan, in theory, cannot fail: but it does demand work. I hope you try it. And I hope you find it's not only the one that worked for Mary Ellen but also the one that works for you.

Joel S. Holger, MD
Minneapolis, Minnesota
30 September 1982

Introduction

I'm in the business of solving problems, and I'm pretty good at what I do. Reading my mail makes me proud. 'Dear Mary Ellen, You helped me solve a problem nobody else could.'

But looking in my mirror brought me down. I was a problem solver with a very big problem – a problem I'd been fighting for years. My weight.

For years I struggled with it. For a while I decided to live with it.

Then, in January 1982, something finally snapped. It was the band on my maternity half-slip, the one I reserved to wear when I was feeling fat. Feeling fat? I *was* fat. Who was I trying to kid? I was telling the salesladies I needed the larger sizes because I'd recently had a baby. The fact was that 'baby' was already reading the newspapers. I hadn't been pregnant in seven years. Now I had had it.

I was ready to start my last diet – the one that worked. It had to be different from all the ones I'd tried before. I found it, and it worked for me. I'd like to share my diet plan, and my story, with you. I think you'll probably find some of it is your story, too. Maybe we can share the same happy ending.

Part One

Help Wanted:
My Story

1. The Gang of One

Among the souvenirs of my childhood, along with a diary into which I had taped my first underarm hair and a letter with Elvis Presley's rubber-stamped signature declining my dinner invitation, is a certificate from the Minnesota Girl Scouts Association. It testifies that in 1957 I sold more Girl Scout cookies than any other girl in the green-uniformed ranks.

Everyone wanted to know how I did it. Here's the true story: I was my own best customer. You know the old line, 'What are little girls made of?' In the winter of 1957, my body composition was probably about half chocolate mint Girl Scout cookies.

Things were never the same after that. Oh, the input varied. You know how the Chinese have the Year of the Dog, the Year of the Dragon, and so forth? I had my years, too. After the Year of the Chocolate Mint Cookies, I had the Year of the Burger and Fries, the Year of the Big Mac, and the Year of the Tuna Melt. The melody would change, but the theme remained the same.

For most of my life, I had a weight problem. Now I don't. I assume if you're reading this book, it's because you have a weight problem, too. Actually, what you have is a fat problem – but I'll explain that later. The point is that you don't feel comfortable with the way you are.

Now, I had a *major* fat problem. Anything over three and a half stone, you have to admit, is a major fat problem. But friends with far less than that to lose tell me that their weight – or their fat – is just as big a problem for them as mine was for me. Carrying around even a few extra pounds, they say, makes them unhappy: their clothes don't feel right and they're very uncomfortable.

Feeling fat affects every stage of your life. Where you work. Where you go on holiday. Whom you end up marrying. How you raise your kids.

My profession has been influenced by my fat. Believe it or not, I have a fairly nice singing voice. And I really believe that if weight hadn't been an obstacle in my life, today I might be a singer. But I always felt: Mary Ellen, you've got to lose the weight before you audition. (Of course, this never stopped Pavarotti, but then they don't write roles like Salome for men.)

You may have had the same attitude yourself: I'm not going to apply for the job of my choice until I'm down to my goal weight. I won't find the man of my dreams until I'm at my goal weight; in fact, I won't even feel comfortable about any guy who's attracted to me now, because after all, what kind of man would like a heavy woman? Now, whether or not this kind of thinking is good for you is a matter of debate, but the point is that in this society, it's very hard to feel good about yourself unless you're lean and fit.

You miss out on an awful lot. After my first book was published and turned out to be a success, the natural thing would have been to treat myself and my family to a little holiday, right? Wrong. Holidays to most people, and to me, mean beaches, and beaches mean bathing suits. Dressed, I was a successful author. In a bathing suit, I was, well, let's put it this way: no beach cover-up manufactured would do the job I wanted.

Actually, I didn't start out in life with a major weight problem. I was a curly-headed baby. People in my family said I looked like a Korean War orphan, but obviously they didn't know what they were talking about because at eight pounds I was a little hefty to fit that description. Granted, that's not what you would call a mammoth child, especially since I was a month overdue, but it's definitely on the large end of the baby scale. I must have enjoyed food right from the beginning because I actually remember first tasting solid foods. It was an experience I can't really explain – remember, it happened before I knew words – but I do remember it was heavenly.

When you're the first child, with a loving, caring mother, you're fed very well. I certainly was. By the time I was eleven, she was already concerned that I might become overweight. I don't believe in kids going on diets. I admire parents who don't nag their kids about weight. The problem will go away if their diets are nutritious and they get exercise. Of course, people are much more conscious of weight than when I was a child. In those days, people thought that kids were cute if they had round cheeks. Now everyone wants to have a low-fat body.

When I began my diet, I set a goal weight of nine and a half stone. That's about fifteen pounds less than Venus de Milo would have weighed, with arms, if she'd been made of flesh instead of stone, according to an article I once read. It's what I weighed at sixteen. I wasn't a beanpole, but I was at a good weight, and I was in shape.

It's generally accepted that your teenage weight, if you weren't a chubbette, is the right weight for you as an adult. That should be your goal weight on this diet. If you can't remember what you weighed, try and check out old medical records. Of course, if you're like most of us who've been dieting for most of our lives, you probably do remember.

My friend Gail, an addicted dieter like me, says that while other people remember where they were on certain important dates, she remembers what she weighed. She knows that when Neil Armstrong landed on the moon she was down to eight and a half stone.

I'm not the only one who has gained weight since my teenage years. The whole country got fatter. I was just doing the American thing. Yes. You may be surprised to hear this, but over the past fifteen years, Americans as a whole have gained weight while eating less.

I'm certainly eating less than I used to. I'm from a Swedish background, and the Swedes eat a pretty hearty diet. My grandfather was a butcher. My mother wrote a little poem that I used to recite.

> My grandfather is a butcher,
> My mother cuts the meat,
> And I am a little rump roast,
> Running down the street.

Ultimately, my grandmother did more of the meat cutting than my mother, since my mother was out working. My grandmother is your typical wonderful, soft, chubby, loving grandmother, and she loved to cook for me and my sister and brother. My favourite of the lunches she prepared was peanut butter and tapioca pudding. After I ate the peanut butter sandwich, I'd have a couple of bowls of pudding. I'd already had my oatmeal and bacon in the morning, of course, and I would be ready for meat and potato and vegetable for dinner.

My grandmother also baked. She made ring doughnuts and yeasted doughnuts, and after they were fried she sprinkled sugar on them. She wouldn't just give us one or two, she'd give us ten. (I'd hide mine so nobody could get them.) But this was a special event. We didn't get dessert and cakes and cookies the way you can today. Cake wasn't a daily item on the menu, it was a weekly treat. If you wanted a cake, you didn't get it in the stores; you made it from scratch. I think if we still had to prepare all our food ourselves, we'd have less of a national weight problem. By the time you get out the pan, beater, flour, and sugar and then discover you're out of vanilla – the urge has probably passed. But you could have eaten a box of cookies in the same amount of time.

Also, have you noticed the national gain in weight is coinciding with the decline in the size of the family? Don't laugh, folks: I think they're related. In the old days, when you divided your cake with the family, you only got one slice. Today, with smaller households, there are three people sharing cakes that used to be divided by six. They're eating twice as much. Also, of course, we didn't have fast foods back then.

What we did have I, was eating. And a lot of it. Still, I wasn't fat, just what they call sturdy. Whatever I ate, I burned up. I never stopped moving. First of all, I don't even remember seeing a school bus when I was a kid. We walked to school, at least three miles a day. After school, we were constantly in the streets playing kick-the-can and baseball. And we had chores. On Saturdays, first we cut the lawns with hand mowers, and then we worked off more energy jumping up and down whenever we stepped in dog-doo, which happened at least once every Saturday. In the fall, we raked leaves into piles, and then we had to jump in the piles, and then we had to rake the leaves all over again. In the winter, which lasts quite a while in Minnesota, we shovelled snow. And after that we had to make a snowman.

We had housekeeping chores, too. When I was growing up, it was my responsibility to iron my own clothes. And that's when I believe my hinting career started. In those days, everything was cotton, and you know how wrinkled cotton gets after it's been laundered. What we did was sprinkle the clothes with water, roll them up, put them in plastic bags, and store them in the refrigerator for a couple of hours. This made the ironing chore much easier.

Well, I had lots of things I would rather do than iron, so sometimes I'd let the ironing go for a couple of days. By the time I got around to my clothes, I'd take them out of the refrigerator and find that they had mildew all over them.

Eventually, the light bulb went off in my head: I'd freeze the clothes. That way I could iron one piece at a time. Of course, we didn't have big freezers in those days, just those little compartments, so there would be several items of my wardrobe stuffed into the spaces where the ice cubes should have been. I was always getting yelled at. 'Mary Ellen, get down there and get your peasant blouse out of the freezer.'

Even when we watched TV we had to move at least a little.

As some of you may remember, in those days you actually had to get up and go over to the set to change the channel. In fact, we didn't watch much TV, and my mother always got rid of the television set in the summer. For some reason, it always managed to go on the blink the week school let out. But we had plenty to do without it. Minnesota is the land of 10,000 lakes, and just four blocks from my home were four of them. They were like private playgrounds for us kids.

For my first twelve years I was a tomboy, involved in everything from climbing trees to stealing apples. Then I discovered boys.

When I became a young teenager, inactivity was voguish. If you were lucky enough to hang around with a group in which somebody had a car, you were really popular. You didn't walk anywhere, and you wouldn't be caught dead on a bike. Only the simps rode their bikes to school.

Looking good ruled out any physical activity – those cotton clothes really wrinkled. We didn't have miracle fibres. Today, you can slip into a pair of polyester trousers in the morning, go stunt riding all day, and they won't show a crease. Back then, the minute you bent over, you were a mess.

And the hairstyles! Hair was tortured into place. You sat under the dryer for hours or you slept in rollers. It's amazing we don't all have permanent furrows in our scalps. I wore medium-sized rollers, which meant my head never got nearer than two inches from the pillow. My best friend set her hair around orange juice cans and slept sitting up. In the morning, you'd take out the rollers and shoot a lot of hairspray over the whole thing. The desired effect was that your hair looked bulletproof. Someone told me my hair looked like a helmet and I took that as a compliment because that meant it must have looked really neat. Anyone who wanted to look good knew you had to move around slowly, so you wouldn't ruin your clothes or disturb your hair.

Until this time, I'd done all right in the gym. I was a great basketball player, and I was good at running and jumping. I'd always felt a little inadequate because I couldn't climb the ropes, but at this point I really started to hate gym class. It was partly because of the group showers. They never upset me so much that I'd hide in my locker, but I was modest, and besides, I was worried about my hair. Here I was at the time of my life when looks are the most important thing in the world, and someone expected me to go to gym class in the second period to do a hundred sit-ups and then get my hair wet on top of it.

It became a big game to get out of going to gym. I was at my most ingenious each spring, when we'd have to do these crazy marathon runs. Mind you, we did not run all winter long, but for some reason the gym teacher thought it would be fun to send us to run four miles the minute she saw a crocus. Of course, today they know this kind of thing could kill a person. But there we were.

I had a few friends who'd already left school, and I called on them for help. I'd start off from the school and go maybe a quarter of a mile. Then my friends would pick me up in someone's beaten-up old convertible with the top down – it was spring after all – and we'd go to Porky's, the local drive-in. We'd all have a Coke and then they'd drop me off a block from school and I'd come in with a fairly reasonable run. I never tried to set any kind of record, because I knew the teacher would figure that one out.

Even though I didn't move around as much when I became a teenager, I still had my former appetite. Gradually I started gaining weight. And I didn't know why. I really, truly, didn't know why. I started cutting back like a typical teenager – going to a café for burger and fries, and a Coke once a day, and then picking all the rest of the day. I never had a major weight problem – but I never got any thinner, either.

So the vicious cycle began.

2. A Fat Madness

I turned on the television one day and two doctors were talking about when diets began. This was an intriguing idea to me, that somebody could pin a date on the whole thing. The experts couldn't narrow it down to a year, but they agreed that fad diets really caught on big in the early 1950s.

I do know that in 1959 a group of friends and I went on the Minneapolis diet. The Minneapolis diet, which we made up, was as follows:

> *Monday*
> Coca-Cola (all you want)
> Pistachio nuts (all you want)

The programme was the same for Tuesday, Wednesday, Thursday, Friday, Saturday, and Sunday. We arrived at pistachio nuts because we decided we were going to eat only one food, so it should be something we liked, and we all liked pistachio nuts.

The Minneapolis diet had two features I always looked for in diets afterwards: 'fast weight loss' and 'eat all you want'. Those were the attractions of the first official diet I went on, something that later became known as Dr Atkins' diet. (When it first appeared, Dr Atkins was probably still a student.) The diet was explained in a book called *Calories Don't Count*, and at the time I believed that. After all, who'd ever seen a calorie?

The *Calories Don't Count* diet was a low carbohydrate diet. From health class I knew that all foods were made of protein, fat or carbohydrate, and I bought a book that gave the carbohydrate count of common foods so I could avoid those that were high in carbohydrates. Still, I had to have my Coca-Cola, even though that used up half my carbohydrate allowance for the day. I starved, and I lost weight. Temporarily.

I went back on that diet when it came out under Dr Atkins' name. I followed Dr Stillman's diet, too. Remember that one? You ate a lot of protein and drank a lot of water. An enormous amount of water. With the obvious results. It was definitely not a diet you'd recommend to someone who, for example, had to stay still for hours as an artist's model.

I liked it because you could eat all the meat you wanted, any kind. My version of the Stillman diet was four pork chops and a gallon of water for dinner. I lost a lot of weight in a single weekend and put it back on the following weekend.

In basic health class, you learned that the body is supposed to be in a state of balance. Everything that goes in and out is supposed to maintain that balance. On the 'miracle' diets, you send the system into a tailspin.

There are many variations of these high protein or high fat, low carbohydrate diets. The secret weapon is ketosis. The theory is that protein molecules are so large and complex that they require more energy to digest, and you can burn extra calories every day just by eating extra protein. Supposedly, you also eventually excrete a by-product of fat metabolism (called ketone bodies) that contains undigested calories. The latest news is that the maximum calories you can excrete in this fashion is only a hundred! Besides, the side effects of these diets are nausea, weakness, lightheadedness and fatigue. You also break down your muscles and weaken your bones, and on top of everything, you get bad breath. I was led to believe that the worse your breath smelled, the more weight you were losing. As if I didn't have enough problems.

I found the vinegar and honey diet floating around somewhere in the sixties. Honey and vinegar are mixed with warm water and a glassful was drunk before each meal. If you've read my other books you know I'm the expert on vinegar. On this diet, the only thing you were guaranteed to lose were your teeth. I didn't stay on it long.

Diets named after foods became very popular about then. I went on all of them. I couldn't wait for the latest women's magazine to come out and tell me about the newest diet. I went on the cottage cheese diet, the apple diet and the grape diet. I even made up one of my own. It was called the sauerkraut diet. I figured that anything tasting that terrible must surely burn off fat. (In those days, I was always hoping to 'burn off' fat. Nobody told me that was a laugh.)

Guess what I found out? There is not a canned food on the market that has more salt in it than sauerkraut. If you know anything about salt, you can imagine that not much weight loss occurred on this diet. I just really hate sauerkraut now.

My girlfriend Melissa had a little more success with her own Arch and Box diet. It was a fast food programme. For one week she took all her meals at McDonald's and Jack in the Box. She'd get up in the morning and drive over to get some Eggs McMuffin and then around lunchtime she'd buy the Box special – burger and fries. Of course, by the end of the week, she'd got pretty tired of burgers and fries, so she'd indirectly cut her calorie intake. She lost five pounds, which she kept off for about five days.

Meanwhile, I was on the grapefruit diet, which meant I drank a lot of grapefruit juice before each meal. (Why? It burned off the fat, of course.) And then you ate one egg, with one slice of bacon. If you had two eggs, you had two slices of bacon. If you had three eggs, you had three slices of bacon. I liked the bacon, but the rules were very clear: if you ate four slices of bacon, you ate four eggs.

Later on, I put two and two together and realized this diet was probably a plot of the American Poultry Association! At the time, I was happy with it, since I lost weight.

By the time I'd gained it back, I'd heard about the Mayo Clinic diet. The Mayo Clinic refused to take the rap for this diet, probably because the diet also originated with the

American Poultry Association. On this diet, you ate two eggs with every meal. Egg yolks, in addition to having 60 calories each, are loaded with cholesterol. (And they don't burn fat.) At the time, I was ignorant of this fact. I thought the diet was great and went on it frequently.

Until, that is, I discovered the Alpine Ski diet. This was similar to the Mayo Clinic diet, but instead of two eggs, you had one. Actually, you had two in the morning and then only one at lunch and one at dinner. Why it was called the Alpine Ski diet I never did figure out. Maybe it was started by the Swiss Poultry Association.

What all these diets had in common was that you were always deprived of something. By 'something', I don't mean obvious no-nos like cake and cookies, but foods that are part of most people's daily routine. On some, you aren't even allowed to eat fruit. I'm not especially fond of fruit, but tell me I can't eat it and I'm ready to kill for strawberries and apples. That's why I never lasted longer than two weeks on any diet.

Naturally, I was attracted to diets that made me think I would not be deprived. Authors had people like me in mind when they started to bring out diet books that made the whole process seem like fun: *The Drinking Man's Diet. Eat, Drink, and Get Thin. Stuff Your Way to Svelteness. Pig Out and Pare Down.* Who do you think was first in line at the bookstore?

I went on every diet ever set in print and several that were passed along in the oral (how appropriate) tradition. For example, the bowl diet invented by my friend Marcia. On the bowl diet, you select your size bowl, and then fill it three times a day with anything you like. But you can only fill it once per meal. The theory is that you might eat ice cream, but you wouldn't put a steak and ice cream in the bowl together. Oh, yeah?

Sandy told me about her three-food diet: select any three foods that have nutritional value and eat them for a week. For one of my foods, I selected 'deli' meats – sausages and pâtés.

I took in so much grease that if I walked barefoot, I tended to skid. Plus I gained weight. Bambi told me *her* magic formula: she made it a rule to eat *only* the specific food she wanted at a particular moment, the more exotic the better. In other words, if she had a yen for veal parmigiana, she had to find a restaurant where it was served. The idea was that the longer it took you to find the food you were in search of, the longer the time period when you weren't eating at all. This was a great idea in the days when exotic foods were harder to get, when the only people who ever heard of, say, Mexican food, were Mexicans. Today, you can get an enchilada in the middle of nowhere.

I was going up and down on these diets for years. If I wasn't gaining weight, I was on a diet. When I dieted, I would read cookbooks. My friends would call and I'd say, 'Can I get back to you? I'm in the middle of a good part.' Eventually I went on a new diet every night, not even waiting for Mondays.

You're going to ask why I didn't go to a doctor. Well, most of them had been unsympathetic to my problem. One told me not to bother to come back until I'd lost twenty pounds. Another greeted me by saying, 'Hmmm. This looks like a beef trust.' Not only did I not like dieting, I didn't want to face a scale.

Then I heard of a doctor who didn't weigh you: he just measured you. He had a thick German accent and I think he was on the run to Argentina when he ran out of money in Minneapolis. He gave daily injections of something extracted, from what I could gather, from the urine of pregnant cows. That alone should have made his patients lose their appetites, but in case they didn't, they were also under strict orders not to eat more than two small portions of meat and vegetables twice a day. No one ate very much under his care, but they all thought the 'magic' injections did the trick.

If I didn't want to see him, I could have gone to Harriet's diet doctor. She'd been with him for fifteen years. He's in

Manhattan, and so is she, but he thought she lived in Philadelphia. That's because he charges $250 a year to see local patients, but only $15 a month to people from out of town. She'd call up and say, 'Hi, doc, it's me, Harriet, calling long distance.' She wanted to have a record of the Liberty Bell ringing in the background until I told her that *it* was cracked, too.

I rejected both these solutions and went to see Alice's diet doctor instead. Well, I didn't actually see him: you had to lose twenty pounds before you could see him. Meanwhile, you were seen by one of his assistants, who sat in small cubicles under laminated plaques of their medical degrees and dispensed large quantities of pills in various colours. In a laughable attempt to appear legitimate, the cubicle doctors took your blood pressure when you came in.

The pills were vitamins and speed. They worked for a while, but soon I became immune to them. Eventually, they just made me eat faster. I also hoovered a lot and called people I hadn't seen for years. When I came off the pills, I found myself booked for numerous lunch dates with people I barely remembered. I also made lists – such as whom I'd invite to a party in five years and the clothes I planned to buy in 1995.

Several years ago, my friend Sandy in Los Angeles invited me to see her doctor. He had his nurse touch the patient, and he touched the nurse, and this way he got emanations that would tell him what foods Sandy was allergic to. If she stopped eating them, he said, she would lose weight. He also told her she would lose weight if she wore green. 'That's crazy,' she told him. 'Try it,' he said.

Before I had the chance to decide whether to fly out and see that one, Sandy found one she swore was even better – a chiropractor-nutritionist, a dual speciality that seemed to be popular in Los Angeles. The doctors out there get crazier the nearer their offices are to the beach, and this one was in Pacific Palisades. He specialized in food allergies, too, and his method involved applying foods to your body to see which ones you are allergic to. The way I pictured it, he'd put fudge on your forearm and asparagus on your abdomen, and from that he'd figure out your story.

He never got to do anything with my abdomen, though. My gynaecologist got there first. He told me I was pregnant.

3. The Hippy Housewife

I was twenty-nine when I became pregnant. I'd been married for six years. I thought of myself as a sweet little June bride, but actually I got married in March. Fortunately, the snow didn't interfere with the ceremony, since I had planned a small wedding. For some reason, I was self-conscious. Though I would eventually do television shows without any anxiety, I felt uncomfortable about having an audience watch me get married. After the ceremony, the wedding party went out to celebrate in a restaurant (where else?).

I weighed about nine stone on our wedding day. I'd got my weight down to even a little lower than that, but the popping of the question seemed destined to be followed by the popping of my seams.

I thought of my high school friend Gail, who each year went off her diet the minute someone asked her to the prom. Once you hook the guy, she explained, it was okay to start eating again.

At my wedding weight, people tell me, I was looking good. I wasn't happy at that weight, though. Until I finished the Help Yourself diet, I can't remember a time when I was happy with my body. I think that's a problem many fat people have. They fall off the diet wagon because they're not satisfied, even when they've reached their goal weight. They don't believe that they're thin enough. I read about a study in which people drew pictures of themselves at the beginning of a diet and then at the end. At the beginning, they always draw themselves looking thinner than they are, and at the end, they draw themselves larger. It takes a while to develop the proper self-image. Anyway there I was, unhappy at nine stone. I vowed that the number on the scale would change. It did – to over eleven stone. I shot up thirty pounds within six months, and there I stayed.

Actually, people tell me I didn't look bad at that weight, either. But no one went so far as to say I looked great. I'm not sure how the weight gain happened. Of course, I was eating a lot of steak. For those who have never tasted it, I just have to tell you a little about pan-fried steak. You take a steak and cut the fat off. Then you pound the steak with a hammer to flatten it. Then you heat a fry pan until it's red hot, throw the fat in till it melts a little, and throw in the steak. (I hope that didn't trigger anybody who's reading this to go right in the kitchen, but I think the recipe's too good not to share. Pass it along to your thin friends.) Anyway, I can probably attribute some of my early marriage weight gain to pan-fried steak.

The weight didn't bother Sherm. He always told me he thought I was attractive. And I want it understood that I'm not putting any guilt trip on him, but often the people you love contribute to your problem. For example, I might have been eating pretty sensibly for the week, then all of a sudden I'd get an urge for ice cream, which is not unreasonable. Even thin people get urges for certain foods. But I was overweight, and you can't really binge when you're overweight and you aren't moving around.

Anyway, Sherm would go up to the store and bring home the ice cream, and he'd have a little dish. I'd have a bowlful. Or two. After eating, I always said, 'Don't ever do that again,' and once he realized what I was talking about, he'd say he wouldn't. Then I would say, 'Now, look, you have to promise me. If I tell you to go over to the White Castle and pick up some burgers, tell me no.'

But I could always talk him into it. Sherm is a normal person. He didn't see anything wrong with eating ice cream or burgers. He thinks like a normal person, in singles, not multiples: one burger, not a sackful, one dish of ice cream, not a bowl.

I remember seeing a Jules Feiffer cartoon that was a strip of panels. Each picture had the same woman in it, and she had the same long face in each. In the first panel she's saying, 'I keep thinking my life would be better if I were married,' and then in the next one, she's saying, 'I would have a better job if I were married,' and 'I would live in a nicer apartment,' and finally, in the next to last one, she's saying, 'I tell myself I would be a happier person if I were married.' And then in the last one, she says, 'And then I remember I *am* married.'

Whether I was married or not, with or without Sherm going out for the burgers or ice cream, I would have had my problem with weight. For years, I tried to solve the problem with one fad diet after another. Then, after six years of marriage, I got the good news: I was pregnant.

We were both thrilled. The baby became the focal point of our lives. I was going to be the perfect mother. I would get plenty of rest. I gave up smoking. Exercise, of course, never entered my mind. Or actually, when it did, I pushed the thought away. I really thought it would be dangerous to the baby.

Some women get morning sickness, and I think they're actually the lucky ones. The others, like me, just get hungry. I did eat the proper food most of the time, but I wasn't just eating for two. I was eating for me, the baby, and a set of quintuplets as well.

I started going to my favourite restaurants and having full-course meals. Things like lamb and beans. And that was just lunch.

Then I started craving Big Macs. As snacks. Not just one Big Mac. Sacks of Macs. There were so many McDonald's bags in the back of my car that they were a fire hazard. Sherm told me he was considering naming the baby Little Mac.

I didn't look pregnant. I mean, my stomach didn't stick out. What happened was my body started filling out around the stomach. I just looked square. I didn't care. I was in seventh heaven when I discovered maternity clothes: the loose-fitting trousers and the big tops were the kind of things I'd been looking for for years.

I didn't want to have to worry about weight. I had deliberately chosen a fat obstetrician. How could she have the nerve to tell me to lose weight? She didn't, and I kept eating, even though the doctor forces you to get on the scales each time you have a prenatal check-up. I couldn't ignore the fact that my weight was soaring.

Well, I'd read all the books about how dangerous it was to get too heavy during pregnancy, and I started to get scared. Up to this point, I hadn't considered myself a binge eater. I considered myself the same as every other woman in America – always dieting to keep from gaining weight. Now I started to feel something was wrong. I was afraid of going off the deep end. Someone recommended that I see a psychiatrist.

The psychiatrist was a man who dealt with addictions – smoking, weight problems, that sort of thing. I can laugh when I look back at this episode in my life, but at the time it wasn't funny. I made an appointment and poured out my story. I didn't leave out a detail – the Big Macs, the lamb, the beans, the works. I did everything but give him the recipes for the stuff I was eating.

When I was finished, this man looked me straight in the eye and told me all these cravings were my way of suppressing my sexual desire. He then went on to tell me that when I got a craving for food, I should try to satisfy the hidden meaning behind that craving. In other words, when I got the urge for two all-beef patties, I should have sex instead. In his opinion, that would solve my problem.

Now folks, my husband worked from 8 a.m. until 5 p.m. and was gone weekends, and I was eating three meals a day plus at least two Big Macs. I also had cravings for food while driving my car, sitting in movies, and strolling through the supermarket. I got so depressed driving home from the doctor's office that I stopped at a McDonald's on the way – this is the truth. I actually went back to see the doctor a second time, because I thought maybe in my pregnant state I had hallucinated the whole thing, but when he gave me the same advice again, I never went back. I think the authorities shut down his operation about a year later.

Meanwhile, I was still eating. I grew out of my maternity clothes. I sat around in my muumuu telephoning friends and trying to get their sympathy.

The nine months went by. Finally, early one morning, my water broke. I was thrilled. I waddled to the car, dashed to the hospital, and checked in. The first thing they did was weigh me. The little mother-to-be weighed thirteen and a half stone.

I was already dilated to three centimetres when the doctor came in to check my stomach. This part is hard to believe, but it's true: she couldn't find the baby.

Needless to say, this made me a little nervous. The doctor was pushing and I was thinking, my God! You mean to tell me I'm not pregnant? Fortunately, a trip to the X-ray department confirmed that indeed a baby was in there. He'd pulled himself into a little ball and scrunched himself all up on one side, probably to make room for all those Big Macs. I'm laughing hysterically as I write this, but it wasn't funny at the time.

Andrew Strelow Pinkham was born six hours later. He weighed a little under six pounds. His mother weighed 193. Yes, folks. I was the first woman in history who didn't lose weight after the delivery. Now, I know there will be a lot of doctors writing to me and telling me this is medically impossible, so I'm going to say that maybe there was some discrepancy between the scale in the check-in and the scale in the maternity ward, but I can tell you whatever it was, the situation didn't do much to lift my postnatal depression.

I was in the hospital for seven days, the oldest mother on the floor. I was twenty-nine. In those days, that was ancient. Since I was in an older and probably more weakened state, I figured it was even more important for me than it was for the other mothers to get my strength back. How? By eating, of course. Besides, I thought eating might cure my post-baby blues, which were severe. I didn't even want visitors.

I told my friends, 'No flowers. Just contributions.' I asked them to send food. I ate everything in those fruit baskets except the shredded cellophane. I even ate the hospital food, that's how depressed I was. Cream soup that looked and smelled like wallpaper paste. Scrambled eggs you could sip through a straw. Ice cream that made noise when you bit into it.

By the time I was ready to go back home, I had started nursing. I was told that could be my saving grace. Not only was it wonderful for the baby, but it would help me lose weight and tone up. The pregnancy and weight gain had made me pretty buxom, and I was concerned at every feeding that I might smother my child. I stopped nursing Andrew at three months and it was the first time the child realized you could see and eat at the same time.

Now that Andrew had his good start in life, it was time for me to begin a new diet, I stocked up on all my favourite diet foods – T-bone steak, pork chops, eggs, butter, blue cheese dressing, and a few vegetables that were low in carbohydrates. Dr Atkins, you almost killed me. I bought your whole premise and with it, half the supermarket's meat and dairy products. I considered those foods – high in calories, high in cholestorol – miracle foods.

I stuck with the diet for a while. Then I started caving in. First I only dreamed about bread. Then I started cheating. An occasional apple. A banana here. A banana there. Still, I was losing weight.

Of course, now I realize that it wasn't what I was or wasn't eating that was causing my weight loss. I was losing weight because I was on the go twenty-four hours a day for the first time in years. Late-night feeds, early-morning feeds, trips to the shops, strolls in the park, changing nappies, doing laundry – I was running in circles. But I hadn't put two and two together yet. I thought it was the miracle food diet that was doing the trick. I went down to eleven stone or so.

Of course, my body wasn't exactly the same. I have a word for those gals who are pregnant. You've got to get that excess baggage off right after the baby's born. Strange things happen to your stomach and your breasts. They never fall exactly back into place again. Then, of course, age itself plays some nasty tricks. Maybe it's not age, exactly, but gravity – gravity and dieting. When you're gaining and losing over and over, something is going to happen to your body, as it did to mine. The cycle was becoming harder to get out of.

I decided to return to work, and after one week on the job I was starting to gain. I was back in the familiar routine. Coffee at home, drive to work, sit four hours, eat lunch, sit some more, drive home, eat dinner, and watch TV. I barely moved. If I had lost the use of my legs, it might have taken me a week or so to discover it.

I was now an addicted dieter. A day wouldn't go by when I wasn't dieting or thinking about dieting. I kept going from eleven stone to thirteen stone plus, at least ten times in the past seven years. My body was a mess. I was all flab. It didn't seem to make any difference what the scale read. I was beginning to look the same at any weight – bloated and flabby. Years before, even at eleven stone, I was looking pretty good. Now, at the same weight, I felt mushy. My body had the tone of a water bed. Dieting had destroyed it.

4. Success Went to My Waistline

The only fat host you've ever seen on television was Alfred Hitchcock, and if you remember, he dealt in the bizarre. He and I were two rare exceptions on the box, where everybody from the quiz show contestants to the soap opera stars is in great shape – physically, anyway.

I started appearing on television to promote my book, *Mary Ellen's Best of Helpful Hints*. It was published by Warner Books in 1979, and like most authors, I came to my publisher's office to discuss publicity. The publicity staff asked me to do a personal appearance tour.

I made my television debut on 'Good Morning, Houston'. For the occasion, I was wearing a pair of blue polyester trousers and a loose smock, which would become my uniform. I thought it made me look like a typical housewife, which it probably did, and I also thought it made me look thinner, which it definitely did not. I did not know either of these things then, or for quite a time afterwards, because I would rather have had major dental work without injections than look at myself on videotape.

At this point in my life, I hadn't seen any pictures of myself for several years. Frank Sinatra didn't avoid photographers any more diligently than I did, and what few snapshots of me existed, I managed to destroy. I was like a member of some primitive tribe who was afraid the photo would capture his soul, but all I was afraid of was that it would capture the roll around my middle. The only still photos of me that exist were taken before I got married.

There are film archives, though. Sherm bought a movie camera to take pictures after Andrew was born and I didn't have the time to splice myself out of all that film. Besides, I figured that if I did, Andrew wouldn't have any pictures at all of himself and his Mum. I left the film alone, but when Sherm showed the movies, I always kept my eyes closed at the scary parts – when I was onscreen.

By the time I started my publicity tour, I weighed over eleven stone. That wasn't the worst I'd been, and it certainly was not the worst I'd get to. Yet, it was enough to make me very self-conscious. People didn't understand how I never worried about what I would *say* on television. Frankly, I was only concerned about my appearance. I always spent much more time preparing for how I was going to look than how I was going to respond to the interviewer. I always knew that my mouth would work, but I didn't know about my face or my body.

That's why I love doing radio. You can have fun and talk and laugh and *nobody can see you*. The first week I was on the road, starting in Houston, I was petrified. Every night I went to bed and I thought, my God, tomorrow I have to get up again and go back on television. The idea was not just frightening, it was awesome.

I think it's interesting that none of my friends ever said anything to me about being fat. Nobody ever sat me down and said, 'Mary Ellen, you've got a problem and it's out of control.' Before then, the conversation would go, 'Mary Ellen, you're such a pretty girl. It would be wonderful if you could take some weight off.' Now my appearance was at the point where no one ever brought the subject up, because I wasn't looking pretty at all.

I looked twenty years older. When I was younger, I was complimented on my eyes constantly. But even these comments stopped, because my cheeks had got so heavy that my eyes started to look very small. My second chin grew a second chin. 'You look a lot like Elizabeth Taylor,' one hairdresser told me. 'She has no neck either.'

When you're fat, you see a fat person on the street and you turn to your friend and say, 'Am I as fat as she is?' If you're with a good friend, generally he or she will want to protect you and tell you you're not, even if you actually are.

The only one who said anything to me about losing weight was a stranger who came up to me in the rug department of a Minneapolis department store to tell me the rug I was looking at was overpriced and also I should go on a diet. She was involved in a dieters' group and it had become a religious experience for her: she was a born-again skinny-Minnie. Now I must admit I resented that. One of the worst nuisances about being overweight is that strangers seem to feel it's an invitation to come up and comment on your appearance – 'You know, you ought to lose some weight' – as if that's something that never occurred to you. Even if you've avoided mirrors the way I did, every once in a while you turn a corner and sneak up on yourself.

Strangers should keep out of it, but I do think good friends should be able to help you without offending you. At the end of my fattest period, before I went on the Help Yourself diet, I had become very demanding and irritable, I was putting myself down constantly, and I was becoming unbearable to be around.

The Mary Ellen everyone knew was disappearing beneath layers of fat. How did I know? People told me – but not until *after* I'd begun to lose the weight. I feel that I'm fortunate that I finally started to diet, but I'm sorry no one felt comfortable helping me face the facts.

I don't think it helps any fat person if, out of the blue, somebody close to her just starts telling her she's fat. I think that could drive a person right into the refrigerator. But a good friend can find the right time, and should. I know that people found it hard to talk to me. Evidently I have a forceful personality, though I think I'm a soft touch and a pushover, and nobody ever had the courage to sit me down and say gently, 'Hey, Mary Ellen, you've got to do something. You look terrible. You're getting bigger by the month.'

And I sure was. I went from being an overweight woman to being an obese woman. The more successful I became, the more my eating got out of control. Now, what you usually hear is that the happier you are, the less likely you'll be fat, because you overeat when you're sad. Yes, I do eat when I'm sad, but I also eat when I'm happy. I eat when I'm bored. I eat when food looks good. And I eat a lot when I'm under stress.

I had felt much more in control of my eating when I was home all day long. I never really succeeded in my struggle to lose weight, but I was always diet-conscious. I skipped breakfast and ate a light lunch, like salad or tuna fish. Dinner was a problem, though. It usually started around the time the early evening news came on TV and wrapped up when Johnny Carson and Ed McMahon were saying good night. On weekends, I looked for a party, and to me partying meant eating and drinking.

Once *Mary Ellen's Best of Helpful Hints* was published, I was on the road a lot. I lived in beautiful hotels, and I won't say that wasn't nice, but I had to deal with the strain of living out of a suitcase and under pressure. I felt a lot of stress. My lifestyle had changed overnight. First, I rationalized: Mary Ellen, in your line of work it isn't important to be thin. I thought that the American housewife could identify with me since I was overweight. I told myself I had a nice home, a good husband, a beautiful child, and a successful career. Maybe, I told myself, you can't expect to have all that *and* a nice trim body.

Of course, one look at Jane Fonda and I should have realized none of that made any sense, but I really believed it. I didn't have much time for self-searching, anyway, on that tour. I went to twenty cities. A twenty-city tour means you are in an aeroplane every day and in a new city every night. You work straight through from Monday to Friday, then you go home, and start again on Sunday.

On the road Mondays and Tuesdays, I drank Perrier water and ate salads, with meat and vegetables in the evening. By Thursday at the latest I was out of control. Certainly part of the reason was that I was lonely.

Television seems to be very glamorous. In reality, you walk into a studio about half an hour before you go on the air, go to make-up, do the show, pack up your gear and leave. You don't spend time socially with the people you're talking to on camera for the simple reason that you have to be on the plane that night and on your way, and they have their own lives to lead. It's all quite impersonal. That's not the fault of the people who host the shows, it's just a fact of life.

After the show, you're alone with your thoughts. There is nobody to give you any feedback on your appearance. How did I look? Did I perform well? What could I do to improve myself? Nobody's there to give you reassurance or provide any kind of companionship when you're on the road alone. Food becomes your friend. You look forward to getting into your room, taking a bath, sitting down and having a meal with your pals – protein, fats, and carbohydrates. The meal becomes the high point that you work towards the whole day. Many people admit that they have had the same experience on tour.

A very famous novelist told me that she was midway through a long series of appearances and feeling terrible about the amount of weight she was gaining. One night, just after she had called room service and asked for a big meal, she thought to herself, what am I doing? I don't need all that food, and none of it is any good for me anyway.

So she called down to room service, identified herself, and asked that her order be cancelled. The reply she got confirmed all her worst feelings about what she was going to eat: 'Sorry, ma'am, we've already put it in the grease.'

I have my own favourite depressing room service story. I ordered a fish dish, and then I changed my mind and told them to forget about the fish and send up a steak instead. (In those days, I didn't realize that fish has fewer calories than steak.)

Whoever took the order must have got a little confused, because when I opened the door for room service a little while later, there were two little vases of flowers, two napkins, two sets of silver, and two dinners on the rolling cart. Do you think I sent one back? Not on your life. Waste not, want not, I figured – it was meant to be, and who'll know?

I called out as if someone was in the bathroom. 'Hurry up, Katie, your steak is getting cold,' and for good measure, 'it's just the way you like it.' Then I tipped the waiter, let him out the door, and sat down and ate both meals. I even changed seats when I ate the second one.

Eventually, I saw how I looked on television. This happened when I began doing three slots a week for 'Good Morning, America'. Some were videotaped from my house in Minneapolis. The truck would roll up and the crew would tape and edit on the spot. I didn't want to look like a complete idiot, so I would sit down and watch while they worked.

To my surprise, I didn't look bad. I came to realize this was because when they taped me in Minneapolis, I was onscreen by myself. I always looked okay alone. But the minute you put me next to a normal-sized person, I looked fat. If I were standing next to a TV host, for example, you would notice that his arms were hanging straight down and mine weren't. My hips pushed them out at an angle. It's a look that comes natural to penguins.

(One host I particularly didn't like standing next to was John Davidson. He's very thin. I secretly considered driving John crazy by paying someone to sneak into his wardrobe closet to take in all his seams a bit so he'd think he was gaining weight.)

Obviously I preferred to be sitting if I wasn't alone on camera. I developed a hint for overweight celebrities. One thing about talk shows, and this rule applies from coast to coast, is that they always have one white host, one black host, and a beige couch. What you do is dress in beige. I mean *entirely* in beige – beige suit, beige dress, beige stockings, beige shoes. That way no one knows where you stop and the couch begins.

Someone said she read this in *Cosmopolitan*, but I've been

using it at parties for years. I'd call the hostess up and ask what colour her sofa was, then dress to match it and get there early enough to plunk down on it. Standing-up parties have never been my favourite for this reason. It's hard to dress to match the wall, particularly if there's wallpaper.

I can admit it now. Underneath those yards of beige, my body was growing fatter and fatter. I was totally out of control. I actually became unconcerned about weight. I decided, 'Look, this is the way you are, and this is the way you're going to stay. Accept it. Go forth. Go forth and hint. Go forth and hint and eat.'

Sandy Hill from 'Good Morning, America' had said to me, when I appeared on the show in the early stages, 'What usually happens when people become successful is that they take off the excess weight. You will. I know you will.' Of course, eventually, she was right.

But I don't want you to think you need to be successful to get yourself to Help Yourself. In fact, you need it the most when you're feeling down. I have a friend who always plunges into her exercises and is especially careful about what she's eating the minute that life threatens to overwhelm her – the dishwasher has broken down, the kids are driving her crazy, her husband has decided to quit his steady job and become a stand-up comic. She says, 'At least I'll have a good body to look forward to.'

When you're fat, you're not happy. My book was doing well and I was making good money. For the first time in my life, I could even afford to go to a health farm. You know what? I was embarrassed to go. I felt there was nowhere I could book into.

I was fat before I had the success with my book and I stayed fat after it took off. The only difference was now I could afford to shop in more expensive fat women's stores.

5. Facing the Fat Facts

January 1982. It had been five years since I stepped on a scale. How time flies. The only gauge I had of the seriousness of my weight problem was the way my clothes fitted. Most of them didn't. I was even growing out of my clothes for the larger woman.

At one point, I'd solved the problem of dressing. I had about twenty-five pairs of black slacks. I'd find a brand that was wonderful – in other words that fitted – and buy five at a time. Then I'd put these together with a blouse with long sleeves and a high collar and a black blazer. Dress it up, dress it down. I was set for every occasion. For a funeral, I'd wear the outfit with a grey man-tailored shirt. For a wedding, I'd have a lacy white blouse under the blazer.

This system helped develop my hinting career, because I had a lot invested in preserving my black trousers. I figured out creative solutions for every crisis: when they started pulling, when they needed reinforcement at the seams. Finally, when I nearly passed out in my black polyester slacks on one particularly hot July day, I decided I'd had enough.

Then I started going to stores that didn't use standard sizes on the clothes. They were marked A, B, C, and D, or 1, 2, 3, and 4. When the zipper doesn't close on a size D, it's not the same as if it doesn't close on a size 20½. I preferred poking my head out of the dressing room to ask if the same blouse came in a size 4 instead of a 42. If it said 'One size fits all' and it didn't, I'd decide the garment was manufactured in one of those countries where the people aren't as large as Americans.

I read in *Vogue* that you don't gain weight in your feet. The people at *Vogue* are obviously not acquainted with serious weight gain. Believe me: even my feet got fat. I wore a size 6 when I was in high school, and I'd gone up to an 8½. I blamed this on the manufacturers, but I couldn't help noticing that other parts of me were getting fat, unusual parts: fingers and earlobes. My friend looped her thumb and index finger around her wrist to see if she was gaining weight. Not only couldn't I get my thumb and finger to meet, but I also didn't like looking at my wrists. I thought I saw the beginnings of stretch marks on them.

Andrew and I had gone to see a revival of Walt Disney's *Cinderella*. Every kid wants to fantasize that he has the most beautiful mother in the world, so when we came out of the movie, I waited expectantly when Andrew asked, 'Ma, guess who you remind me of in that movie.'

'Who, Andrew?'

'You remind me of that fat little mouse that laughed a lot.' Andrew immediately realized he'd hurt my feelings, because he tried to turn his comment into a compliment. I almost wished he had said I reminded him of the wicked stepmother. At least she was thin.

Once again, I vowed I had to do something. The first step would be to confront my body, at this point a stranger to me. I had taken to undressing in the dark. If somehow my head and body got separated, I didn't think I could have picked my body out of a line-up.

There was a time when I used to love to look at my reflection in store windows, but now I didn't even have a full-length mirror in my house. The only mirror I used was on my dressing table, and it was a small one, so I could only see myself from the lips up.

When you get really fat, things you think about a lot are your face and your eye make-up and your hair, not your body. It doesn't exist. Then all of a sudden one day you find yourself walking down the street and you see a fat woman walking towards you and you realize you're walking towards a mirror. Some sane part of me knew I had to see myself as I really looked. Not only did I not want to confront the mirror, but I also knew that once I did I'd convince myself that the mirror was exaggerating the situation.

I started thinking about how when I appeared on television, I'd ask the hosts to give me the 'thin camera' and they'd always say 'Are you kidding? I keep that one on me.' But, of course, the camera doesn't lie. A photograph is incriminating evidence. I decided I should have someone come over and take pictures of me.

The morning the photographer came, I was in a good mood. I decided it would be a fun and games day. I went upstairs and stepped into my maternity trousers. Yup, I was still wearing them. I kept them to wear when I was fattest, and by this time they were really comfortable because they were good and stretched out. I put on a blouse and tucked it in. Of course, fat people never wear anything tucked in, except maybe a napkin, so that was a sign I really meant business.

On television I'd learned something about how to pose for pictures. Most heavy people do. Keeping your chin up has real meaning for fat people posing for the camera. They also try to keep their arms up – anything to counter the effects of gravity. Hanging from a trapeze would be good. The major thing is never to face the camera square on; always be photographed in three-quarter shots. Well, I decided I would do this right, so I really did face the camera. Side *and* front, back and front, sitting on a chair, skirt in, low heels. You've seen those before and after shots in every magazine. The gal looks like a real frump in the before shots – no make-up, messy hair and no smile. I did some like that, and I also did some in full make-up. I had a really good time, even posing for some gag shots stuffing food in my face.

When the photographs were developed, I can't explain how I felt. I couldn't believe that I had been walking the streets looking like that and no one had made a citizen's arrest: I was defacing the landscape. It was absolutely mindboggling. I couldn't delude myself that it had been a bad day, because in the photographs I'd taken in full make-up I looked about as good as I could look.

Normally I would have headed straight for the refrigerator, but with the image of those photos in mind, I was too depressed even to do that. There's not a doctor on earth who could have told me to lose weight and convince me to do it, but those photos did the trick.

I looked back at my dieting history. So far, nothing had worked. What could I do differently this time?

Most diet books tell you to have a physical examination before you go on a diet. Physical examination means you get on a scale, of course. The one at home was gathering dust. I had had a couple of check-ups after Andrew was born, but I'd always tell the doctor not to tell me what I weighed. One of the things I'd rather have done than weigh myself was go to war. I truly believe I would rather have died of some disease than get on a scale. I was that obsessed.

But I happened to talk to a gal who told me that she'd had a major weight problem, and the doctor had discovered it was all because she had an underactive thyroid. He'd given her some pills and bingo! She lost two and a half stone. Well, of course I thought this was sensational news. I was thoroughly convinced I had a thyroid problem. All I had to do was go to the doctor and get the thyroid pills and I'd be Miss America in six months.

I made an appointment.

The day before I went, I didn't eat. The night before I went, I didn't sleep. I took a laxative. If I'd had some diuretics, I'd have taken a few of those. I was hoping the doctor wouldn't absolutely have to weigh me, but I knew it wasn't likely. Even the dermatologists weigh you. I used to say I'm here for my skin, not my waist, but those nurses would get me on the scales before I knew what was happening. When I got to this doctor, it was clear the nurse meant business, too.

Of course, I don't think a nurse's task is an easy one. If

I were a nurse, I'd see to it that all fat patients were sedated before they weighed in. I'm probably typical. First I gave her a hard time about my height. When I was in high school, I considered myself a medium-boned woman of average height, but the fatter I got, the more I liked to think of myself as large-boned and tall. The nurse had the nerve to tell me I was only five foot five. I indicated that I had my doubts about her competence.

She had her revenge, of course, by weighing me. She just kept moving those counterweights to the right. Finally she got the scales to balance. What was amazing to me was that lights didn't go off, bands didn't march in and no 'tilt' signs started flashing. No one fainted. I *nearly* did. I weighed fourteen and a half stone. What helped me keep my composure was that the nurse who was weighing me looked as if she were good for well over seventeen stone herself.

Okay, so that was the news. I was more than five stone overweight. Even so, just by going to the doctor's office and facing the scale, I felt as though a big burden had been taken off my shoulders. It was still around my stomach, of course. But being in the doctor's office was just another sign to me that I meant business, that I'd just taken another big step. Who really cares what the nurse thought? Being there was a signal to me that I had some self-esteem left.

I hadn't met the doctor at this point. The doctors never weigh you in, of course. They give all the dirty work to nurses. Eventually he walked in, washed his hands, and then gave me his full attention.

'Well, well, well,' he said. 'What do we have here?'

They always say that. 'Well, well, well. What do we have here?' At fourteen and a half stone, it was awfully hard to miss what he had there. I told him what I thought he had: a person with a weight problem who needed her blood pressure checked. A person who, I advised him, probably had a thyroid problem.

The doctor took a few tests and called me back to his office. The tests had all come back negative. I was in good health.

The doctor said, specifically, 'You are in good health.' I was never so disappointed in my life. 'You are in good health,' he repeated, peering over his glasses, 'but you are fat.' I hoped he wasn't charging me a lot for his diagnosis.

My blood pressure was a bit high, he said, and my heart rate was, too, but he felt they would come down if I lost some weight.

What I really wanted was a thyroid pill. I was convinced that my thyroid was a mess. It's not as if I hadn't made several serious stabs at losing weight. Amazingly, as I look back, I realize that he never asked me if I exercised. He just gave me a 1500-calorie-a-day diet and gave me a lecture telling me to stick to it. In other words, he had no real solution for me.

My worst moment was when my glance fell on my folder lying open on his desk. It said 'obese'. 'Obese' is a word that even if you don't know the language you would stay away from. It's not a word I've ever been fond of, particularly as applied to myself. I was devastated. I would rather have served a prison sentence than be called 'obese'.

Before I got through the front door of the office, I started rationalizing. I had been through a rough experience, so I needed food. I drove out of the doctor's parking lot and into the restaurant's next door. I ordered a salad and diet soda, which I suppose meant something – I could have asked for a burger, fries, and a Coke – but the point is that I was still using food as a crutch. When I faced a problem, it was the first thing I thought of.

I was very desperate. I started thinking about a stomach stapling or intestinal bypass. I can't tell you exactly how they're done, but surgically the doctor fixes up your insides so you don't keep enough food in your system to gain weight. It sounded good to me. I called various doctors in the area requesting either process, but I was told you had to be at least seven stone overweight to be considered for the procedure. I wasn't quite seven stone overweight, so for one brief moment I considered eating my way up to qualify.

Fortunately, before I began working my way through Minneapolis' McDonald's franchises, I read something pretty horrifying: stomach staples pop and bypasses become ineffective. Somehow, within two years of the operation, most patients gain the weight back. Plus, thanks to whatever the doctors have done to your insides, you put in quite a few hours in the ladies' room, if you know what I mean. That put me off. In fact, this was one of the reasons I'd never tried the Beverly Hills diet, which is heavy on roughage. I can think of nicer ways to spend my free time.

So I did the only thing I knew how to do. I started to crash diet. I deprived myself completely. I ate almost nothing all day, slept about ten hours, and barely moved. I was like a dry alcoholic who has given up drinking but continues to show the same obnoxious personality traits. They're belligerent and demanding. They think I'm a good guy, you're a bad guy, I'm deprived, I'm not drinking, the world owes me something. They haven't changed their attitude about living. The only difference is they're not sitting around with a glass of booze in their hands.

That's how I was acting. I felt deprived. I felt angry. Why me, God? I thought. Why should I weigh fourteen and a half stone? I'm a great person. What have I done to deserve this? And the more you think like this, the more you want to eat. Alcoholics have the same experience, only they want to drink.

The longer this went on, the more I was convinced that something was truly wrong, and I was determined to do something about it. I had to find a diet that I could live with. I didn't know what it would be, but I knew I couldn't go back to doing anything I had done in the past. My first thought was to fast, to check into a hospital and live on liquid protein; but I had done similar things in the past and I knew they didn't work.

Remember Scarlett O'Hara out in her garden, looking at the sky and vowing she'd never go hungry again? Well, I went outside to my garden and vowed I'd never be hungry and fat at the same time again. There had to be some explanation for what was going wrong with my body, and I decided if it took me to the day I died, I was going to find out what it was and get the fat off in the process.

It made me feel better to have made this decision, but I had to find somebody who'd help me find the answers.

Thank goodness, I got flu.

6. What's Up, Doc?

After my experience with Dr 1500-Calories-a-Day, I made a vow to stay away from anyone dressed in white unless he sold ice cream. Then I came down with flu. For a while I was in heaven – after all, I was losing weight.

After a few days, my friends and loved ones advised me that my coughing and wheezing and whooping and monopolizing of the loo were rapidly becoming a pain in the neck. Besides, I had a very important business meeting coming up. One of the fellows I worked with insisted that I should see his physician, Dr Joel Holger.

I like my doctors a little overweight with grey hair. Dr Joel was blond and looked exactly like a ski instructor, minus the parka. That, combined with the fact that he seemed unusually nice, led me to wonder if he was a bona fide doctor, but he had the right certificates hanging up in his office, the pharmacy honoured his prescription without any question, and he cured my flu, so I guessed he was.

I actually liked him. Every once in a while we'd run into each other socially, and I got to the point where I'd drop by his office so we could have coffee and talk a little, which for me is the equivalent of Red Riding Hood paying a social call on the wolf. I kept expecting him to give me what I thought of as 'the doctor lecture' about my weight, but he never made it an issue. I even tested him. If we were out and everyone was having pizza, I'd take a slice just to see if he'd say, 'Put that down, Mary Ellen, you're ready to explode,' but he never did. The truth is that I'd already made a commitment to myself and was attempting to control my weight. I wasn't gaining – but I wasn't losing, either. Dr Joel was aware of this because I'd mentioned it in passing, but we didn't discuss it right away. Then, little by little, I started expressing my concern.

I discovered that Dr Joel, who specializes in internal medicine, was very interested in nutrition, and from time to time he'd mention some fact passed on by friends who were doing research in the field. He told me that there were a lot of new discoveries about weight control that might be important and helpful to me, and finally he suggested that maybe we should get together and talk about it sometime. I agreed. For one thing, I trusted him. For another, I had run out of diets. I was eating very little most days, and the weight wasn't coming off.

The day we had our first discussion, I was sitting on Dr Joel's couch. Actually I was sitting on part of his couch. In those days, at my fattest, I always removed the back cushion on sofas. That left more room for my body.

Once I was nice and comfortable, we decided to start at the beginning. Dr Joel asked me to describe the diets I'd gone on in chronological order. I was really proud as the minutes passed by. I calculated I'd been on over seventy diets. Dr Joel had already developed writer's cramp by the time I was up to 1971.

'Sorry,' he said when we were finished. 'I have to tell you you're an addict – a diet addict.' Of course, he said, I wasn't the only one. The majority of American women are addicted dieters.

I knew that. Dieting isn't just a means to an end any more, it's the fashion. If you're dieting, that means you care about how you look. If you're not dieting, you're a schlep. Even the kids know this. My friend's little three-year-old son refused to wear a white suit she'd bought him. Why? He came up with the excuse he'd heard from the grown-ups: 'It makes me feel fat.' My own son Andrew, who hasn't got an ounce to spare anywhere on his body, sometimes asks, 'Ma, when can I go on a diet?'

Today, right after they say, 'How are you?' people don't

ask 'What's new?' or 'How're things?' like they used to. They say, 'You're looking thin,' which means good. I do it myself. I did a guest appearance on a show with Orson Welles once and I told him *he* looked thin.

'How are you?' means hello. 'Have a good day' is a form of saying goodbye. When people say it, I usually want to jump off a balcony, but they say it anyway. The whole rest of the conversation gets squeezed in between 'How are you? You're looking thin' and 'Have a good day.' Only when you're walking away do they turn to a friend and say, 'Boy, she's looking fat.'

And of course I was, which is the reason I'd finally come to Dr Joel. After he took my history, he really endeared himself to me by not weighing me right away. First, he spent some time explaining why every one of the fad diets that I went on was a nutritional disaster. 'You're kidding,' was my first reaction. 'Even that nice lady who tells me to stuff my face with pineapple is talking through her hat?'

On top of that, he told me that there is no food that burns fat. Was I disappointed! I felt like the kid who learned that there is no Easter Bunny and no Santa Claus. On the same night.

Worse news. A lot of these diets are truly dangerous. Calories-don't-count diets – the ones that are low in carbohydrates and high in fat – strain your kidneys. Others are lacking in bulk, or vitamin C, vitamin A or potassium. Really strict diets, especially when they lack protein, are very dangerous. If you don't take in enough food to meet your body's energy requirements, the body breaks down its own tissue – even tissue from vital organs like your heart. (What's the difference between a vulture and a fad diet? The vulture waits until you're dead before it eats your heart out.)

As fast as I could come up with some other diet I'd been on, Dr Joel would tell me how it could kill me. Still, that wasn't the worst news he delivered about dieting, and if you're a fat person, you'll know what I mean.

The worst news was that *dieting helps make you fat*.

Dr Joel explained it all scientifically, but I have to confess I missed most of what he was saying the first time around. All I could think of was that nobody had told me the truth. All those ladies' magazines and all those diet books I'd read, and all those doctors I'd seen talking on chat shows weren't really giving me the whole story. I never believed everything I read in the papers or all the claims in the commercials, but I believed everybody who came out with a new miracle diet. Now it turned out that I shouldn't have. No fad diet helped me do anything but get fatter.

It seems that there are two main causes for what Dr Joel insisted on calling 'obesity'. I told him that was one of my least favourite words, but he said that 'overweight' was – for reasons he'd soon explain – not really accurate.

One reason is primary hyperphagia, which in plain English means overeating. The other is primary obesity, which in simple terms is a tendency to get fat. We primary obesity types, the scientists now think, may react to long-term rigid dieting by increasing our fat production.

This made sense to me. Sure, I overeat some things. Who doesn't? Even the thinnest people I know sometimes eat dessert when they're not really hungry for it. But it seemed as if I were cutting down on my food over the years and still getting fatter and fatter. It wasn't just a lack of willpower that kept me fat, Dr Joel was saying, it was actually the diets I went on.

There seems to be some evidence that every one of us has what authors William Bennett, MD, and Joel Gurin describe in *The Dieter's Dilemma* as a setpoint – a weight our bodies go to unless we're restricting our calories. That's why some of us are always battling the same ten pounds and why even though others get fat, they don't go all the way up to circus-fat-lady size. In my teens, my setpoint was around nine and a half stone. My setpoint, in postpregnancy, was thirteen and a half stone. No matter how I dieted, I always wound up back there if I stopped watching what I was eating.

Dieting, it turns out, can't lower the setpoint. We fat

people have been on diets constantly. And the result of constant dieting is to lower the rate at which you burn food – your basal metabolism.

Dr Joel explained that the human body is designed for survival. It was designed so we could go for very long periods without food, in the days when there were no twenty-four-hour supermarkets and all-night cafés. And the most efficient way to store food, he further explained, is in fat because it's concentrated. Fat has more calories per pound than carbohydrates or protein; for example, a tablespoon of butter (fat) is more fattening than a tablespoon of rice (carbohydrate) or fish (protein).

Our bodies are very clever about saving up the fat stores. When you diet and lower your food intake, your body lowers its fuel-burning rate so the food will burn more slowly. Your body thinks, we must be stranded on a desert island somewhere. Less food is coming in. So we'd better burn our supplies more slowly. And this happens even if your body has plenty of fat already tucked away for an emergency. It's as if your body has landed on a desert island but doesn't realize that the *Queen Elizabeth* is washed up alongside it.

Anyway, pretty soon you stop dieting, and you're off the island and back into McDonald's. Your body doesn't know this right away (news is slow to travel from the mainland), so it continues to burn food more slowly.

You're taking in the same amount of food as you did before you began dieting, but your body is burning that food more slowly. You're gaining weight. If you happen to be taking in a little extra, in a post-diet splurge, you not only gain back what you lose, but a few extra pounds besides. How long your basal metabolism rate is set off-kilter is not certain – but it is long enough to permit a weight gain.

As if that weren't bad enough, the new, heavier you is composed of a higher proportion of fat than when your diet began. If you lose twenty pounds, ten is probably water, five lean muscle, and five fat. What you regain is ten pounds of water and ten of fat, assuming you don't exercise.

The more muscle there is in your body, the faster you burn calories, even at rest, just in the simple acts of breathing and circulating blood. On the other hand, fat tissue uses up calories much more slowly. The new, fatter you needs even less calories than before you dieted, but you probably haven't cut your usual calorie intake, have you? This is a second reason for weight gain.

I was a textbook case. My metabolism had gone haywire, my body composition was too high in fat, and with each new diet I was struggling harder to lose weight. The worst part of it was that my setpoint, which had been around nine and a half stone, had moved up to thirteen and a half stone and, like inflation, seemed to be going higher with no end in sight.

Could I move it back down?

Could I get my metabolism operating like a normal person's?

Could Mary Ellen Pinkham, a gal from the Mid-west, find happiness as a thin person?

Yes. Dr Joel finally delivered a piece of good news. He told me that all the evidence seemed to indicate that you can improve your metabolic rate. He had a theory about it, and he asked me if I'd like to be a guinea pig (which I suggested wasn't the most tactful phrase). A test case? What the heck, I told him. I'd done whatever every crackpot who wore a stethoscope told me to do and followed the advice of a few crackpots without them. Now, someone I trusted wanted me to try his method. How could I refuse? I had nothing to lose but my weight.

Part of his theory involved reducing my calorie intake. A diet, in other words. But there was a new twist. Over the course of the diet, as I lost weight, Dr Joel would slowly add to my daily calories. He was certain that his system would permit me to ultimately take in hundreds of calories a day more than I was now eating and stabilize at a normal weight. To break the crash and binge syndrome, it was important that I get my metabolism used to a normally high intake.

I had been either dieting or gaining weight for as long as

I could remember. There was no in-between for me. And none of the fad diets I'd ever been on ever paid much attention to what happened once the diet was over. The idea that I could, at some point, eat like a normal person was very appealing.

A nutritionist would work out the details of the diet, and Dr Joel thought I should help her set the ground rules. I also wanted a very strict plan. Nutritionists think structured diets are a bad idea. They say that people want to 'rebel' against them, and structured diets don't teach you how to select food for yourself. But I wasn't ready to make my own choices. For one thing, I really didn't know much about calorie values. Besides, we addicted dieters are so used to rigid rules that we need and like them. Our past dieting history has turned us into robots. Tell us what to eat, how much, what time, and we'll do it. We're incapable of making choices because we're afraid of making the wrong ones, and if we do, the miracle – fast weight loss – won't happen. Dr Joel and I compromised: I would start with a strict plan, then go on an unstructured one once I felt capable of taking control.

I also thought the nutritionist should give me a shopping list for the strict plan part of the diet, and I asked for other considerations.

1. Keep me out of the supermarket. I only wanted to shop once a week.
2. Keep me out of the kitchen. If I wasn't supposed to spend a lot of time eating, I didn't want to spend a lot of time cooking (and tasting).
3. Don't plan for any leftovers. I am a member of the Clean Plate Club Hall of Fame. I have eaten meals on behalf of the starving peoples of every nation. I am unable to prepare a recipe that serves four and eat only a quarter of it. If a diet calls for half a cantaloupe, I worry about what will become of the other half, so I eat it. But if I know I'm supposed to save it for a meal later in the week, I will.

We agreed that the diet would begin on 31 January. I would go to Dr Joel's office for instructions about the non-diet part of his plan, which he hadn't yet explained to me.

I had long since got past the point of postponing diets to Monday mornings. At this point in my life, I planned on going on diets every day. In honour of the occasion, I'd often have a big blowout the night before. Mr friend LizBeth actually started the tradition of Farewell to Food celebrations. She had refined the system so that she would actually have a theme to her eating. I remember Ebony and Ivory Eve, Mint Monday, and White-on-White Night, which was my favourite. It started with potato soup, and continued with turkey on white bread, followed by rice pudding and sponge cake with vanilla ice cream, marshmallow topping and blanched almonds.

Typically, after eating on a Farewell to Food night, I would go to sleep and have a deprivation dream. An ice-cream vendor would refuse to sell me Chipwiches. All the hot dog stands in New York burned down.

But on 30 January 1982, I dreamed that I was at a party. Gloria Vanderbilt was offering me a tray of hors d'oeuvres, and she was saying, 'You're much too thin.'

I knew this time would be different.

7. The Moving Experience

Dr Joel was ready for me on 31 January. He had even removed the back cushion from his sofa so I could settle in comfortably.

We had worked out the details of the diet. Now he was going to explain the other part of the programme. 'You're going to exercise,' he said.

Exercise? That was the secret weapon he was going to use? Visions appeared before me. Sit-ups. Push-ups. Me in a leotard. Richard Simmons ordering me to do one hundred leg-lifts. I told Dr Joel he had to be kidding.

I was well acquainted with the argument that stepping up physical activity is an ineffective way to lose weight. I remember reading a magazine article about twenty years ago that said in order to burn off a pound of fat, you had to walk from Mexico to California. Or maybe it said you had to walk ten miles. Whatever it was, it seemed a long way to me.

That article cinched it. I thought, what is this? You have to put in that much effort to burn off a pound of fat?

So from the time I was in my teens, I looked for diets that discouraged physical activity. Most of them did. They never actually said exercise was forbidden, but they were always accompanied by little charts that told you you had to cha-cha for ten hours straight and then chop down the Yellowstone National Forest to work off the calories in an apple. I reminded Dr Joel of all of this.

Then he told me a couple of things. The newest research shows that exercise might be helpful in speeding up your entire fuel-burning mechanism. In other words, scientists now think that when you exercise, you don't only burn up

61

a set number of calories, but also you speed up your rate of burning. And this effect might last for as long as twenty-four hours after you have exercised.

Also, and especially important for someone like me, there is a good chance that exercise can reverse the damage done by dieting. Dr Joel reminded me that as a result of going on my very first diet, I'd lost muscle. It's harder to break down fat than muscle, so when I cut down my calorie intake, my body went to the most easily available source of extra calories – my lean muscle mass. When I regained weight, I gained fat, because you only regain muscle if you exercise, which I had not done.

That's why Dr Joel told me I shouldn't think of myself as overweight, but overfat. There are some people who weigh exactly what they should on the charts, but the fat content of their body is too high in proportion to the lean muscle mass. You've seen them, with their little pot bellies and flabby arms. Ideally, women's bodies should be composed of about 22 per cent fat. I didn't know what per cent fat I was, but I had a suspicion that if I got too near a flame, I'd melt.

Dr Joel said that by exercising, you can change the proportion of fat and muscle in your body. The larger the proportion of muscle to fat in your body, the more calories your body uses at all times. Muscle uses more calories than fat just to go through the processes of daily life. An athlete in good shape uses more calories to breathe than a thin person does. Standing around, looking good, Chris Evert Lloyd burns up more calories than I did running around the block. It didn't seem fair.

Yet Dr Joel's explanation made sense to me. In my opinion, I was moving around quite a bit, but my body just wasn't burning the calories properly. What about shopping? I was doing a lot of shopping. Didn't moving around from store to store count for anything? Look how thin Jackie Onassis is. I was shopping all the time and it wasn't doing a thing for my body.

Also, I did walk around the lake once or twice a month.

Of course I didn't enjoy it. I dreaded it. Every step I took was agony. I knew it was important to give your body a real workout every once in a while, and I thought my bi-weekly walks were good for me. As a matter of fact, I figured they were especially good since they hurt. Physical activity in my mind was equated with pain. The theory was, 'No pain, no gain.'

Dr Joel asked me to write down as best I could what I had done for the past couple of days. I had just come back from a trip to New York, and I had spent the day before this one going about my regular work routine. I'd spent two very busy days running from appointment to appointment. Well, 'running' wasn't exactly accurate. Dr Joel asked how I got from place to place. Of course I went by cab in New York or by car in Minneapolis. I almost never went on foot. The automobile is the American way. Travelling by car is very patriotic, I told Dr Joel, since it supports the car industry.

Dr Joel said that my heart was in the right place even if it was buried under layers of fat. He suggested that if I really felt the car industry needed my support, I could make a donation to the Chrysler company. Then he told me an amazing piece of information. He had read that the activity level for Americans had fallen so dramatically that the average person would easily have gained twenty pounds in the last twenty years if he had not also cut down his food intake.

When I thought about that a little, I realized I had seen it happening firsthand in the difference between my mother's generation and my own. I don't remember my mother ever going to exercise class or taking any kind of regular exercise. Yet she and her friends never really had a weight problem, and they all ate three square meals a day. (Plus, I remember a lot of coffee breaks in between meals, with lots of real cream and sugar and homemade pastry on the table.) Why? They were truly physical beings.

We all lived in two- or three-storey houses, and that meant a lot of running up and down. And every day had its share of demanding household chores. When our mothers did a wash, they had to hang the clothes on the line to dry and then they had to iron them. When was the last time anyone I knew ironed an hour a day – or an hour a week?

We didn't have wall-to-wall carpeting. We had rugs, and even though we did have vacuum cleaners – I'm not that ancient – I remember my grandmother taking the rugs out once a month and throwing them over the clotheslines and beating the heck out of them.

We walked to the stores. You didn't make a weekly trip to the supermarket, you walked to the grocery store whenever you needed things, and you walked to the butcher and the baker and the hardware store. Everybody walked. I had to admit that if I compared that shopping to my couple of spins around the air-conditioned mall, I really wasn't getting much exercise.

It's funny that during my childhood you never saw a grown-up at the lake. Oh, once in a while the other kids and I would spot what we considered a weirdo taking a run, but the lake was mostly just ours. Today, there are bicycle paths, jogging paths, and hiking paths, and a lot of people are on them, but most of us are just kidding ourselves. We may go to the exercise class once a week, but let's face it: we're sedentary.

Dr Joel didn't want me to do any exercise other than walking. Somehow, 'walking' didn't really seem like 'exercise' to me. For 'exercise', you need equipment. My usual pattern on the few occasions when I decided I might get some exercise was to outfit myself for it. (A bonus in this plan was that I could put off doing the exercise until I got to the sporting goods store.) Buying the outfits was the only truly pleasurable part of exercising for me. I think that dated back to my teenage years, when I had positive feelings about my school gym uniform. It had a blue bottom with a white top, and we had our names embroidered on the top. My mother was a great seamstress and she could really embroider. She did my name in very decorative embroidery, and since it was Mary Ellen Higginbotham, it stretched out very nicely across the top of my pocket clear around my back, and really stood out. (Of course, that goes to show how thin I was. In recent years I could have crammed the whole name between my pocket and my underarm.)

I had not only become convinced that exercise was relatively pointless in weight control, but I also was having a harder time finding the clothes in my size, with the possible exception of rugger shirts. Besides, I didn't think I cut a really impressive figure. You don't look like a Wimbledon challenger in a size 44 tennis skirt. As for exercise class, the word 'tights' has new meaning when they're stretched around thighs that are the same size a waist is supposed to be. My thinking was, I can't show up at exercise class until I lose weight. I'll look better and move better then, and I won't embarrass myself as much. The truth is that a lot of fat people are very agile, but they don't want to expose themselves in public, which is a very sad thing.

At one point, I was going to take up jogging. There was one very attractive feature to jogging that I could see. The clothing has elastic waists. I got myself a nice blue velour outfit and blue shoes and blue socks and a blue knit cap and blue sunglasses. I even got myself a jogging bra, that's how serious I was. I felt terrific. The only thing that didn't work out was the jogging itself. (Fortunately, the outfit wasn't a complete waste. I wore it to a Hallowe'en party and told everyone I'd come as the Pacific Ocean.)

Dr Joel made it clear he was not telling me to jog. I was supposed to walk. He showed me how to test my pulse to see if my pace was brisk enough. But the most important thing was that I was to do it no less than five times a week and never skip two days in a row. Of course, you don't have to be a doctor to know that going out and playing a couple of exhausting sets of tennis just a couple of times a year wins you the key to Heart Attack City. But it turns out that regular exercise is not only safer, but it also increases the benefit of the exercise. According to the estimates, exercising four or five times a week is three times as effective as exercising only three times a week; and exercise once or twice a week has little effect at all.

Dr Joel also made me take my measurements. I was in perfect proportion – exactly ten inches too much of me in every key spot. I asked Dr Joel if by any chance he had any suggestions – since I was going to be exercising anyway – for doing something about my cellulite. You don't have cellulite, he said. So, I figured, maybe I'm being too hard on myself. Maybe my hips are fine. No, Dr Joel said, there is indeed something on your hips, but it's just fat, in another shape. There is no such thing as cellulite.

And there is no such thing as spot-reducing. (I felt really bad when I thought of the hours I'd wasted walking my hips along the floor. I couldn't say I'd miss doing it, though.)

Dr Joel pointed out that if spot-reducing really worked, gum chewers wouldn't have double chins and typists would always have skinny fingers. He explained further that if you do a lot of sit-ups, your stomach muscles will be in great shape, but if you're still too fat, they'll be buried under a layer of marshmallow.

It seems that walking exercises the largest sets of muscles in your body, and when you exercise large sets of muscles, fat is drawn from all over your body. My thighs and all the other parts of my body that were too fat would slim down without any exercise other than walking. It sounded too good to be true, but I committed myself to go through with Dr Joel's plan.

On 1 February, I started the diet and exercise programme. I knew I'd have more trouble with the exercising than the diet. After all, I'd been on diets before. Of course, I'd never dieted and exercised together. I wouldn't have considered it possible. Everyone knows you need extra food when you exert yourself. Doubling the day's calorie intake for every five minutes of exercise seemed like a good rule of thumb to me in the past.

But I was determined to stick to this programme. Dr Joel

had cleverly started me with a pretty modest exercise programme. Part of my whole way of life is to think that if a little of something is good, a lot is better. If someone tells me to exercise for five minutes, then I think I should go out and do thirty. Of course, the next day I'm so worn out I don't want to do any. Dr Joel understood this, so he told me to start by walking twenty minutes, and twenty minutes only.

On 1 February, I got up and walked for twenty minutes and then I came back and ate my breakfast. In those twenty minutes, just walking briskly, measuring my pulse rate the way I was supposed to, I actually worked up a little sweat.

The next day I decided to do my twenty minutes at lunchtime, so I drove myself over to the lake and walked around for twenty minutes, then drove myself back to the office.

This went on for a week. I was doing my walking, but it was like taking medicine. I hated it. I never experienced any pain, because a twenty-minute walk just didn't do that, but the twenty minutes seemed like an hour. I was doing it because I had to.

I sat down and took a critical look and realized I was going out of my way to do the walking. In the morning, I forced myself to go ten minutes from my house and then turn around and come back. I wasn't going anywhere, or looking at anything, and I was taking the same path every day. At lunchtime, I drove for two miles to take my little twenty-minute spin. It was ridiculous.

I said to myself, 'Mary Ellen, you're the kind of person who needs a purpose to what you're doing. Some people would enjoy walking aimlessly, but you don't. So give yourself a destination.' That Sunday I walked to church. I was up to thirty minutes by then, and that got me there. I felt so good that after church was over, I turned around and walked home. I started walking to visit my friends. I started walking to the grocery store.

Then I started looking at my other alternatives. I decided that I could try walking to work. It was exactly the right distance for an hour's walk. I treated myself to a cassette player with headsets, got some great tapes, and off I went. I was my own car. And the more I walked myself around, the more I enjoyed it.

Friends who were runners used to tell me they couldn't stand to miss a day. 'I've got to get out and run. I don't feel good when I haven't moved,' they'd tell me, and I couldn't understand this. The amazing thing was that in a matter of two weeks of exercising every single day, my body started to crave exercise, too.

I can't say there weren't setbacks, but I just kept plugging away. The only thing that was really important was getting out of the front door. Once I'd done that, I found I could always keep going. One day I found myself whistling as I walked. For a change, I wasn't feeling sorry for myself; I was actually enjoying the walk. That was the day I really got hooked – and it was only a month into the programme.

An added reward that came along was the wonderful times walking gave me with my son. I had been really inactive before and now Andrew started looking forward to going out with me. Before, our activities had always centred around food. Maybe we'd go out to a movie first, but the big treat was always going out for what I euphemistically referred to as 'a bite' to eat. My little boy did not like sitting in restaurants. He wanted to be out doing something, and once he found out that I would be going along with him, he said, 'Any time, any day, Mum. You can wake me up early. I'll go with you.' He hopped on his bike and rode back and forth while I walked alongside him.

There isn't one thing about the walking that hasn't made me feel good. I've probably moved more since January of this year than I have since I was nineteen. I don't roll out of bed any more, I spring out. New verbs have entered my life: skip, run. In New York, I used to take cab rides that were so short the meter didn't even jump. Now what's jumping is me. I don't use the excuse that I can't walk because I'm wearing high heels; I keep my tennis shoes in a very nice canvas carryall that I take everywhere.

I used to take my legs for granted. Now, when I walk, I feel them carry me along. Sometimes I look down and watch them move. I think about how they're getting firmer and stronger with every step. I imagine that with each one, I'm leaving a little bit of fat behind.

And then, midway through the diet, those same legs betrayed me. They took me out for a binge.

8. When the Compliments Stop

Picture it. I'm at the halfway point. A scant eleven and a half stone. Somewhat less than a Green Bay Packer, quite a bit more than a Russian gymnast, and holding. I haven't lost an ounce in two weeks. Am I mad? Will I get my revenge? Of course. I'll eat something. The only question is what. I'm in New York, an eater's paradise.

I put on a beltless dress and hit the streets, just another New Yorker striding along with a purpose. Mine happens to be cake.

I turn into the first likely spot, one of those places with baked goods on revolving stands in the window. The cakes are very tall, nearly as tall as the hairdo of the hostess who seats me. The waiter hands me the menu and I turn directly to the last page. It's called 'The Grand Finale'. A whole page of desserts. I go for something simple: a slice of chocolate fudge cake à la mode with a glass of skim milk on the side. What's cake without milk?

The order is there in no time. As the waiter puts it in front of me, he gives me a little smile. 'Enjoy, gorgeous,' he says.

Yes. He said 'gorgeous'. I'm saved. I want to jump up and kiss him. I'm not hungry any more. I leave the cake and milk untouched, put a large tip beside it, pay the bill and leave.

Until not too long ago, there was always someone offering a psychological explanation for bingeing. It was the result of unresolved conflicts in my life or a dieting depression that just overpowered my willpower. Then the American Psychological Association said being fat was a physical problem only – not a psychological one. That pleased me: I never much liked the idea that I was fat because I was some kind of psychological mess.

Of course, in the long run, it didn't matter. I was dieting and exercising to get my metabolism working again, and no matter what caused me to binge, I had to find a way to stop it.

As usual, my first few days on the programme had been a breeze. Sure, I was eating less, and walking more, than I wanted to, but the beginning of a diet is like the beginning of a love affair. You feel proud and optimistic, and you have someone to daydream about all the time: your future self.

Within a very few days, between the walking and the dieting, I had lost six pounds. I thought, 'Boy, I'm in control. I have several good days behind me.' I wanted to speed things up. My urge was to start fasting. I felt like Mother Theresa, full of goodwill towards myself and others, cleansed, and a little fragile, which at over fourteen stone is some indication of what a wonderful imagination I have. Dr Joel reminded me that if I crashed, I wouldn't be taking off fat anyway. Most of what you lose when you crash is just water. He advised me to sit back and relax and follow the programme.

But I was on such a high, I was so sure I was in control, that I couldn't wait for a chance to test myself. People were starting to invite me out to dinner. I was still on the first few days of the programme, the very restricted part, but I thought, 'I can handle this,' and off I went.

I found myself with my hand in the breadbasket, then dipping my breadsticks into the butter, and eventually I realized then and there I wasn't ready to be out eating. The evening turned out to be a positive experience, though, because I found I was able to ignore the slip and just start right back on the programme. Besides, the diet menus were good and eating three meals a day not only satisfied me, it was a novelty.

Staying on the programme became even a little easier as soon as I began to get the compliments from my husband and friends. I loved the attention. It was terrific. All I wanted to talk about was how wonderful I was starting to look, how great I felt and what I was and wasn't eating. If a conversation wasn't about me, I felt that at least it should be led by me.

My friend Ian invented a little imaginary event he called the Boring Olympics. There were a variety of competitions, such as Speed Boring and Long-distance Boring. He told me that Mary Ellen and her diet and her walking were taking top honours in all of them. I was becoming the Number One World Class bore.

Enough already, I told myself. Lives are going on, the seasons are changing, Liz is having marital problems, there's a new heir to the throne of England, there are other subjects to talk about than how loose your waistband is. Put things in perspective. People want to talk about more than how you look and your diet programme. Enjoy the compliments and shut up.

Then came the really rough period. The compliments did stop. That made it very hard for me. I was working hard to stay on the programme, my weight had plateaued so I didn't even get any satisfaction out of stepping on the scale, and my diet and I had lost the Number One spot on the Hot Topic Parade. That's what led me to the cake.

When the waiter helped snap me out of my mood, I realized that I needed a lot of attention to help keep me going. If people keep telling you how great you look, not only does it make you feel good, but you're also a lot less likely to pile extra helpings on your plate.

I made a point of getting out among friends. In the past, when I'd go on a crash diet, often I'd lock myself up, go to bed early, do anything possible to keep myself away from humanity and food. Well, you can hibernate for maybe two weeks if you're a social creature like I am. I knew I'd be on this diet a lot longer than two weeks, so I had to find a way to be social without over-indulging.

After my slip at the dinner party, I did limit my activities in the very beginning, but after a couple of weeks, the diet had become part of my routine. Besides, Dr Joel insisted that I kept a book and wrote down everything I ate all day, together with the calorie count. This seemed especially silly to me in the beginning, when I was following the diet he gave me exactly, but it was a little like writing out the multiplication tables when you're a kid. By the time I'd written down '1 medium-sized baked potato – 100 calories' a few times, I knew the calorie count without thinking. I had a better idea of what damage I'd do if I took a little taste of this and that. I'll never forget the day I was looking through the calorie book and I noticed that Roquefort dressing had 100 calories. Per *tablespoon*. I wanted to call all my friends to warn them. I didn't know where to write to complain.

I had never been one of those people who went to a party for the food rather than the conversation, but I did find it was a good idea if I positioned myself a little farther than usual from the cocktail and buffet tables.

When discussion of my weight wore thin before I did, I decided to find something else to fall back on. I decided to change my style. Working on my appearance would give me something to look at instead of the blasted scale.

At my fattest, I was always perfectly groomed. My hair was perfect, the make-up was flawless. I had long nails and dark polish and I wouldn't be caught dead in flat shoes. I felt thinner being taller.

If I went on a trip, the excess baggage I carried wasn't just around my waist. When you're fat, you need to take a lot of clothes with you. In the first place, your things wrinkle faster than thin people's. In the second, you never really feel comfortable in anything and you somehow think that changing into another outfit will make you feel thinner, which of course it won't. In the third place, you have to be prepared for every emergency. You can't get a pair of queen-sized beige sandalfoot pantyhose in every corner of the globe. If you're in Alaska and someone finds an indoor, heated swimming-pool, you want to have your skirted bathing suit with the built-in bra along, just in case no one can lend you one.

I wanted to create attention, so I went for the opposite of what people expected of me. Since I was a little thinner, I felt secure enough to pare down in every department. I went to the beauty shop and had my hair cut off and shaped into one of those styles you aren't supposed to bother with. Off came the nail polish and half the nail tips. The silk dresses went to the Salvation Army. I adopted a disguise: tennis shoes and slacks, shirts with the tails tucked in. No one would believe it was me.

Then I started to change my look every time I started getting sick of myself, mostly with make-up and hairstyles. I bought a couple of inexpensive wigs to make the change more dramatic. One week I was carefree, the next careerwoman, and then I went back to glamorous. I kept up the routine for months. My friends started calling me Sybil, but the trick kept me going.

About a month after I had started the diet, I felt secure enough to get rid of all my fat clothes. A lot of them had the original price tags on them. (But not the size tags: I always removed those immediately.) In the group were smaller-sized clothes that I had intended to wear after I lost weight. They were now too large.

There came a point when not a single thing in my closet fitted. Everything was too big. I treated myself to some new clothes. I know it's a bit of a waste, but I don't think you should keep running around in size 20s when you are down to 16s. Buy yourself a couple of pairs of inexpensive trousers and shirts that fit to wear in the interim, and remind yourself of the money you've saved by cutting down on the eating.

I was continuing to cook for my family during the diet. In the past, I had had a lot of trouble keeping myself from sticking my finger into the cookpot and sampling. Now that had become less of a problem. I was making a conscious effort not to do that, and I wasn't cooking the kinds of dishes that lend themselves to that kind of sampling. You don't stick your finger into a grilled fillet of fish.

Even after I went off the rigidly structured part of the programme, I liked to plan my meals in advance, particularly the dinners. I got out a pad and paper and my calorie counter and I figured out what I was going to eat for the week. It made my shopping easier, of course.

In the beginning, I repeated a lot of the foods I'd eaten during the first two weeks, mostly because the nutritionist Dr Joel was working with had made up some delicious menus. As I started feeling more comfortable about making intelligent choices, I branched out.

My family actually liked the new system. We had been eating a lot of the same foods over and over again, with a lot of beef as the main course. My tendency was to switch over to chicken, since that was a good low-calorie food, but the nutritionist suggested I vary the menu for my sake and the family's. So I found some new options. One night it would be prawns, the next night something else. Sherm and Andrew told me they'd be looking forward to what we were having next.

Fortunately, I didn't have the problem my friends told me about. Their husbands just didn't want to eat the kinds of foods their wives prepared when they were on diets. Of course, my first reaction is that if the guy won't give up his mashed potatoes and deep-fried chicken for you, leave him. Doesn't he know that both of you will benefit when you're looking better? Also, if you're healthier you're probably going to be around a lot longer, and if he really cares about you, he should be all for that, too.

But I can't say I didn't have my problems with being sabotaged. It happens in marriages where the wife or husband has a weight problem and the thin partner says, 'Let's go and eat.' He knows it makes you happy. I don't think the partner is doing it to be mean or malicious. There's a lot of love involved. 'Hey, you've done a good job now, and you've lost some weight, so eat the ice cream.'

The same thing happened when we went to my mother's house. Sundays at my mother's have always been an event for me, my sister, and two brothers. We just let it all hang out, and we did a good job of eating. This particular Sunday I remember was Mother's Day, and there were several kinds of cake on the table and I was going to have a little portion. It really did satisfy me to have just a couple of forkfuls. Suddenly I heard, 'Oh, Mary Ellen, you should have a nice piece. It's Mother's Day.'

One's reaction is to get angry, until you realize you're being coaxed by somebody who believes the cake will make you feel good. Sure it will. For as long as it's in your mouth. But now you have to start dealing with the long term.

That Sunday, I posed for a lot of pictures, which I had been doing all along. Pictures serve two very important purposes: they help show you that you are getting thinner, and that you aren't thin yet. Those Mother's Day photos were a kind of landmark occasion for me, because I posed next to a lot of normal-sized people. And yet when I looked at the photos, for the first time the people in them didn't seem to have limbs like Olive Oyl compared to mine.

I had seen a woman on television who lost ten stone on a natural food diet. The show pictured her at her top weight and then at her goal weight. At the end, she didn't look as good as you would think, because her body was not toned; she hadn't done any exercise. She looked like a smaller version of a fat person, with the same roly-poly arms, just smaller dimensions. She wasn't taking up as much space, but she looked exactly the same. But I could see that wasn't happening to me. I felt very good.

I had to keep that image in my mind to keep going when I had a last major near-setback, about three-quarters of the way to goal. I met some friends in a restaurant who hadn't seen me for a very long time. I heard a lot of 'Hey, Mary Ellen, I don't believe it,' and 'You look like a movie star.' And then, halfway through lunch, someone said, 'You know, you're really different. You're not fun any more.'

I thought, do I have to decide if I'm going to be fun or pretty? Because if it came down to it, I'd rather have a good time than look in the mirror. When I got down to goal, of course, I realized I could do both. At the same time.

9. Fat No More

I am a firm believer that fat is the best method of birth control. Not until I lost weight did I start getting patted on the fanny again instead of on the back. I see myself in a completely different light now. I love to wear negligees, for instance. I used to hate them. Well, of course I did. It's hard to breathe deeply with passion when you're afraid the seams are about to go. Forget what you know about nylon being so strong they make parachutes out of it. There wasn't a nightgown built for the strain I put on it.

As I write this, I'm at my goal weight of around nine stone. I've stabilized at it, and it seems to be the right weight for me. Now, I know there will be some anorexic type on the telly telling you and me that people five foot five should weigh around seven stone, but I won't buy that. No, I'm not reed thin, but I'm in good shape. I think I look pretty good with my clothes on.

I go shopping for dresses and I don't need to ask a saleslady what makes me look good. I know when I'm looking good. Whenever the saleslady shows me a dress that looks as if you could fill it with foam pellets and make a beanbag chair out of it, I say, 'Get that out of here.' I want everything to be fitted. I absolutely will not wear another sack dress again, whether it's in fashion or not. I don't want to feel as if I have to cover myself up.

On the other hand, I'm not about to sign up for the Miss Nude America competition, either. I have my war wounds, my stretch marks. And sometimes that's hard for me to deal with. Let's face it, there probably isn't a person in America who wouldn't like to fiddle around with his or her proportions. Take a look at a line-up of dancers. These are people who are working out their bodies every day, who are in the best shape it's possible to be in. Yet some of them are a little too busty, or they have rib cages that are too big, or hips that are too wide or their waists don't go in the way a waist should go. There are very few Bo Dereks or Farrah Fawcetts out there.

Even if you suspect that you're contoured more like a ginger ale bottle than an hourglass, there's no reason to work yourself up from the six-ounce bottle to the two-litre size. Even if you believe the setpoint theory, I think it's hard to accept the idea that thirteen and a half stone is the setpoint that Nature intended for anyone under six feet tall.

When appearances are doled out, we each get a different colour hair, eyes, skin – the whole bit. We even get a normal weight – normal, that is, for the individual. Even if yours doesn't put you in the fashion model category, so what? There aren't enough jobs to keep that many of us busy as fashion models. Maybe you got a little extra in the personality department, or you're a great mother.

Weight's only part of who you are. If you get yours down from a definitely obese fourteen to eleven stone or from eleven down to ten, be grateful and proud of what you've accomplished. Keep on the diet, stick with the walking. Your shape will definitely get better, whether or not you knock off more poundage. It's not how many pounds you weigh, anyway – it's whether those pounds are fat or lean muscle that determines how you look.

The important thing about getting on the Help Yourself programme is that it's for life. You may see me somewhere eating a burger and fries, but you won't see me let a week go by without exercising for at least five days. I have had weekends when I've eaten to excess – not pigging out like in the old days, but eating more than I needed. When I was going on and off my fad diets, if I ate a little extra, my weight would shoot up five or six pounds. Now, it goes up just a little, and as soon as I notice that weight gain, I do something about it. I still find it difficult not to try and fast it off, but I have made a commitment to my body never to do that again. I do as Dr Joel suggests: I cut back 400 calories, and keep walking, and that always corrects the situation within a couple of days.

I also keep a daily record of what I've eaten even when I'm overdoing it. It doesn't seem like a nuisance any more. It's part of my daily routine, like brushing my teeth, and thanks to all the practice I had looking up calories, I'm now pretty familiar with the information. I can gauge the count of almost everything I eat and keep myself in check. Of course, now that my metabolism is working like a normal person's, I can pretty much eat what I like, and that's a real pleasure.

I was amazed to discover that I had actually worn out two pairs of walking shoes. I've worn out high heels before – with all that weight on them, I'm surprised I didn't grind them right down into stumps – but I can't get over the walking shoes. I'm thinking of having them bronzed to use as planters or doorstops. They'll be souvenirs.

My other souvenirs are in the photo album. I look at those photographs, and I have a hard time realizing that person was me. I think of myself as a thin person now; I've stopped making those fat jokes that I was the butt of.

When I look at those pictures, I can't help thinking, how did I let myself go? but I try not to blame myself. I tried to control my weight, but like most of the public, I was a victim of deception and hype dished out by a lot of so-called diet experts.

I got sick of hearing about weight loss and talking about it. Find another hobby, I said to myself. But no matter where I went, someone would be talking about losing weight, and then somebody else would beam down with some other 'miracle diet' she heard about or read about or some gypsy in the street thrust in her hands.

They have a lot of different names, but I call them the Fool Yourself diets. They have about as much basis in reality as any other science fiction. Remember the movie *Invasion of the Body Snatchers?* Well, I was waiting for the invasion of the fat snatchers. Sorry, folks. They're not coming.

So I felt it was time somebody wrote a book that told the truth. No magic formula. No gimmicks. Just the assurance that it works. It takes a lot of effort, but I learned to Help Myself. And you can learn to Help Yourself, too.

Part Two

Help Yourself:
the Programme

10. If You Really Want to Help Yourself, Read This Part

I'm now going to explain why the Help Yourself programme works and why you should follow it (though, of course, you should check with your doctor before you start).

If you're like me, you want to rush past this section and get right to the diet. You don't want to be educated. You want to be thinner. Forget it. The diet is the least important part of this programme. The diet alone is not what's going to make you lean and fit. That will happen only if you stay on the full programme, and the only way you'll be really convinced that it's important to stay on it is to read what comes next. Then you'll know why the Help Yourself programme will get that fat off and keep it off – and why any scheme that doesn't combine a well-balanced food plan with an exercise programme (with a little bit of habit changing) will not.

It doesn't matter who comes on to the scene next – some guy telling you to dine on tree bark because it's high in fibre or a woman plugging the Miss Universe I Love the Galaxy diet or yet another doctor swearing on his stethoscope that you can lose weight following his magic plan that involves combining foods that rhyme – save your money. If you go on another one of those crazy diets, you're going to fail. Oh, you may lose a few pounds, but, ultimately, you'll gain them back. Ninety-eight per cent of dieters do. Then you'll feel guilty, get depressed, and start eating – and keep right on until the next crackpot scheme comes out.

Let me tell you the truth, which most of the diet book authors in the past have not. If any diet you go on isn't based on the principles I'm about to explain, it can't work.

Here's Why You're Likely to Be Fat
- It may be genetic
- It may be physiological

First the Good News
It's not your fault you're fat. Some people think fat people are just self-indulgent slobs who have no willpower. Most of the fat people I know display an amazing amount of willpower each time they start a new diet; they may eventually fail, but they make some awfully good tries. Other people think it's a mental problem: fat people are mental wrecks who head for the refrigerator every time they have a mood swing.

In 1980, the American Psychological Association got you off the hook. They issued an announcement that obesity is a physical disorder; it is not linked to a psychological problem. You may sometimes eat for emotional reasons – even thin people do – but that's okay. It's a problem, but you don't need years of therapy to uncover some dark spot in your psyche that's drawing you towards chocolate. Congratulations, sort of. You're not nuts; you're just fat. Why did you overeat so much that you got fat?

Your Genes Made You Do It
You're not used to thinking of your weight as a trait like your hair or your skin, but it is. Forty per cent of children who have one overweight parent will have a weight problem themselves. Eighty per cent of children with two overweight parents will. One reason for this may be that you pick up your parents' habit of overeating. But there also seems to be a genetic influence on your weight.

Being fat is always connected with how much you exercise. Researchers at Harvard noticed that even in infancy, there is a difference in how much individuals move. Babies who moved the most were the least likely to be overweight, even though they also ate the most. Babies who ate the least and moved the least were fattest. (I thought it was also interesting that babies of rat mothers who exercised while pregnant had a lot more muscle fibres in their bodies than other rat babies. If your mother didn't exercise, here's something else you can blame on her.)

Also, how fat you are is determined both by how many fat cells you have and how large they are. How many you have seems to be determined by heredity. You acquire most of the fat cell supply during your first two years, with an additional supply coming in at adolescence. (Pimples and fat: no wonder the teen years are so miserable.) Some unfortunate people have both a lot of fat cells and large fat cells. While you can shrink fat cells, as I did, you can never reduce the number, and having a lot means you tend to be a fat person.

In addition, some people's bodies have more of a special ingredient that helps them burn their food faster than you and I. It's called brown fat, and if you haven't heard of brown fat it's because scientists have only confirmed that it exists in adults within the last three years. (It exists in newborns to help maintain body temperature.) It's not something you'd notice anyway, since the largest deposit in your body is between your shoulder blades and it takes a thermogram to find it. Nobody yet knows what determines how much brown fat you have. Perhaps it's genetic. One theory postulates that it can be increased during a particular period of overfeeding during infancy. Back off from those baby food jars anyway: if you start overfeeding junior at the wrong period during infancy, he'll get an excess of the plain old white fat we all know and loathe.

Studies of people who matched in every respect (such as body size, amount of activity, and food intake) have shown that one might lose as much as twice as much body heat as the other during metabolism, and by losing that heat they burn off extra calories. In other words, people with a lot of brown fat can eat twice as much as other people – and not gain weight. Conversely, a lack of brown fat might make you gain weight easily – but that's not been proven yet.

Finally, there may be something wrong with your body's

regulatory system that explains why you and the guy next to you have eaten the same amount but he's ready to quit and you aren't. Your stomach and blood sugar may be sending the message 'enough already', but for reasons scientists can't yet explain, it isn't getting through to your brain. A Cornell University Medical College study turned up a substance produced in the small intestine that may signal when you've had enough to eat. Obese rats have less of this substance than non-obese rats, and the same may be true in humans.

Even a specific craving for carbohydrates, which seems to affect women more than men, may have a chemical explanation. In most people, a brain chemical called serotonin increases after a small amount of carbohydrates are eaten, and the person stops craving more. In some fat people, serotonin activity stays too low.

Your Body May Have a Naturally High Weight

Some experts believe that your body has a natural weight or setpoint, which they describe as the weight your body reaches when you aren't counting calories. You may want to weigh nine stone, but your body's trying to get to eleven stone. William Bennett, MD, and Joel Gurin, who outlined this theory in *The Dieter's Dilemma*, explain that dieting is like pulling against a spring: you struggle to lose weight while your body struggles to keep it on. Perhaps this problem is linked to a substance called lipoprotein lipase (LPL). Obese people have more LPL in their blood. LPL levels go down during dieting, but return to high levels during maintenance.

Remedies

What does this mean to you? Until there's a pill that can reverse the effect of whatever it is in your body that made you move too little, produce too many fat cells or too little brown fat, or causes chemical imbalances, you've got a problem. Just like you've got a problem with hair that's mousy brown or skin that's too dry. But you change your hair colour if you don't like it, and you do something about your skin. And if you're fat, there's no reason to stay at home crying into your bag of cookies. Even the setpoint theorists say you can change your setpoint. You *can* do something about your weight problem. It must be done over a period of time, and it will be harder for you than the rest of the (thin) world. But *it can be done*. I'm living proof.

Why Fad Diets Do You In

- No fad diet is based on the critical 'energy equation'.
- Fad diets make your system sluggish and promote eventual weight *gain*.
- Fad diets increase the amount of fat in your body – even if you lose weight.
- The more fat there is on your body, the harder it is to get fit and lean.
- Your 'weight problem' is actually a 'fat problem' and you can even be a *thin* fat person.

Input and Outgo

The energy you derive from the food you put into your body (input) and the energy you spend in keeping your body alive and moving (outgo) are the two parts of the 'energy equation' that determine your weight.

Fad diets concentrate your attention on input – what you do or don't eat. You eat grapefruit, or eggs, or cottage cheese or you may even count calories, and presto! The weight will come off. This approach makes the assumption that everyone's body works the same, which, of course, is not true.

Think of a car. How much fuel it requires doesn't depend on the size or style of the car but on the efficiency of the engine. Human beings are living things, so every part of them needs food for energy – that's why a fifteen-stone rugby player needs more food than a seven-stone secretary. But even among people of the same size, there is a variation in how much a body stores and how much it burns up.

Common sense tells you that to lose weight, you must take

in less food than you need. Even 'eat all you want' diets, which always restrict you to a set list of foods, are based on reduced calorie intake; it's been found that no matter what you're eating on a restricted plan, you soon get bored and eat less than usual.

Fad diets concentrate on reduced input, but never concern themselves with the other half of the energy equation: how you burn off that energy. The way to do it is through exercise. I know you've heard about how long you have to walk to burn off the calories in one apple, but, as I will explain, exercise does a great deal more than use up a certain number of calories.

Fad Dieting Made Your Problem Worse

If you have a genetic tendency to be fat, you probably went on your first diet around the time you started noticing the opposite sex. That's when you first got into trouble. Here's how:

You lost lean muscle. Let's say you lost twenty pounds. About half of it was water. Sorry, folks, but that's the truth. About five pounds was fat. And five pounds was healthy, lean muscle. More about the consequences of that later.

You slowed down your metabolic rate. Your metabolic rate is the rate at which you use energy (food you have eaten or food you stored as fat) and generate heat (a by-product of the process of using energy). When you're tested to find your *basal* metabolic rate, that's the rate at which you're burning food while at rest.

Dr Joel explained to me that when there's a drop in food intake, the body, which resists weight loss because it wants to keep itself intact, starts to burn the food more slowly. The effect lasts for several weeks, possibly longer. No one knows for sure.

End-of-the-diet weight gain. By taking in less than your body needs to maintain itself, you cause your body to become fatigued. At the end of this diet, two things happen:

One: the fatigue and depression of dieting almost

automatically cause you to crave more food and then to overeat.

Two: your metabolism is still working at a lower rate, yet you're eating as much or possibly more than when you began the diet. Experimenters starved laboratory rats for a while, then put them back on their normal diet. During the first week of eating normally, they gained more than twenty times the weight of animals who had been fed the same amount without being starved first. (There is an additional theory that this may also be linked to levels of LPL, the substance I mentioned on page 88.) When I found out about this, it was the first time I'd ever felt badly for a rat.

This is why any fat loss programme should get your metabolism working properly by gradually increasing the amount of food you take in as you lose weight. Instead of being trained to work more slowly as you eat less (that's what happened on a fad diet), on the Help Yourself programme, your metabolism is slowly adjusted to working harder and harder. When you've reached goal, it's 'set' to burn off the calories you're taking in.

Fat Makes You Fatter

I have mentioned that on a fad diet you lose lean muscle. If you don't exercise, you replace that lean muscle with fat. Here's what that means to your body:

Fat tissue is, for the most part, inactive. It carries on some metabolic processes, but at a low rate. It uses few calories. Lean tissue, on the other hand, is active muscle, and it does use calories. The more of your body that is made up of muscle, the more calories you use up in doing everything from breathing to walking. And vice versa.

If you regained your weight after the fad diet, you probably continued to eat the same amount as before you dieted. Even if the scale stayed the same, since you didn't exercise, your body contained a higher percentage of fat than before, so it actually needed less food. The result was you got fatter.

When you're fat, your body doesn't burn fats properly. Everything you eat, you will remember from your health classes, is made up of protein, carbohydrates or fats. When you need energy, your body gets it by burning carbohydrates first and turning them into glucose. Since only a relatively small amount of glucose is kept on hand in your body (after a very short time it is put into storage in the liver) the body quickly uses it up and then dips into its fat stores.

Humans and animals store any excess food as fats. Camels, who store fat in their humps, convert the fat to water during their long desert trips, which inspired me to a poem:

> The camel stores his fat in humps.
> Yours is in unsightly bumps.
> The camel's fat helps quench his thirst.
> Yours just makes you look your worst.

The unfair fact is that people who are fat do not give up their stores of fat easily, the way lean and fit people do. If you're in good shape, you can dip into your fat stores readily. If you're not, you cannot. You need energy, though, so you get hungry. That's why fat people often want to eat after exercise and thin people do not.

Eventually, the fat stores of unfit people will break down, but only over a long period of time. Fat bodies were designed to exist during times of famine; but in a civilization of abundance, like the United States, they just get fatter.

Being fat predisposes you to getting fatter. The metabolic processes of obese people are altered. Their fat cells store more fat more easily than those of thin people. The problem you have just gets – pardon the expression – larger.

The Scales Don't Tell the Whole Story

Like most people, I tactfully refer to my 'weight' problem. Enough of this beating around the bush. The problem is fat. There are even *thin* fat people running around. Dressed, they look like skinny people. Undressed, you'll be relieved to know, they look like you and I. You've seen them. They weigh what the charts say they should, but they have narrow shoulders, no waist, and thick thighs – any or all of the above. They keep their weight down by eating very little.

Many women claim that they eat hardly anything and they're still not lean and fit, and that's true. Most American women eat less than 1600 calories a day, which is about right if you weight eight and a half stone – ideally, you sustain your weight by eating about 14 calories per pound – yet most American women weigh more than eight stone. They're not in shape, and they've wrecked their body's system through fad dieting. Ideally, a woman's body should be composed of about 22 per cent fat (men's should be 17 per cent) and yet many are higher – up to 45 per cent. The only real way to know what per cent fat you're made of is by having some rather sophisticated testing done, but you can get an idea by doing a little pinch test.

This might be easier if you ask a friend to do it. I hope you can find a close and supportive friend. There are four spots to test:

a. Take a vertical pinch from the back of your arm midway between your shoulder and elbow.
b. Take a horizontal pinch about an inch below your waist and an inch to the right of your belly button.
c. Take a diagonal pinch just above your hipbone.
d. Take a vertical pinch from the front of your upper thigh.

If you have any doubts about whether you're fat, pinch a skinny friend and compare yourself to her. Or take my word for it: if you've got an inch in at least two of those places, you're too fat. Or, if you absolutely want to know the worst, you can ask your doctor to measure these skinfolds (that's what they're called in the medical biz).

When I heard that men's metabolic rates were higher than women's, I didn't think it was fair. I even considered having a sex-change operation. Then someone pointed out that men burn their food faster because they have less fat on their bodies.

Increasing the percentage of body muscle, and decreasing the percentage of fat as a result, is vital in a programme that will make you lean and fit. The only way that can be done is through exercise. That's why Dr Joel made exercise such an important and necessary part of the Help Yourself plan.

Why the Help Yourself Plan Is the Only Type That Can Work

- What a successful plan must combine
- Why not eating a well-balanced diet is dangerous
- Why eating several times a day helps you lose weight
- Why exercise is critical to a fat loss programme
- Why it's necessary to change your habits

How a Fat Loss Programme Must Work

A plan that works must include a diet that modifies your intake; exercise, to change the regulators of the outgo; and a set of guidelines to help you change your eating habits.

The Eating Plan Must Start with a Well-balanced Diet

A government committee studying nutrition reported that a person should take in a daily mixture of 15–20 per cent protein, 50–65 per cent carbohydrates, and 20–30 per cent fats. You should avoid excessive sugar and fats. You should also eat four times a day and not skip a meal – not even breakfast. We know how many times you have heard all this. But have you ever had an explanation?

Eating the proper balance keeps you from getting hungry and also keeps you healthy. As you now know, your body first uses the carbohydrates you have eaten, and then, when it goes through the limited store of these, it goes to the fats for fuel. Fats are broken down last, and they help give you that full feeling that prevents you from overeating. So they should be included on any diet in modest amounts.

If you aren't taking in enough carbohydrates when you eat, you interfere with the normal sequence. If you run out of carbohydrates quickly, your body will start breaking down protein before it goes to fat. The protein being used comes from muscle, which is meant to be part of your body's structure, not a source of energy. If your body is desperate, it will break down even organs, like the heart muscle. When you lose weight rapidly, as you do in most fad diets, that is always an indication that muscle is being lost instead of fat. (Fat contains many more calories per pound than muscle; it takes longer to lose a pound of fat than muscle. Also, muscle, unlike fat, is associated with a lot of water, which leaves your body along with the muscle.) Experimenters put some animals on fad diets and others on sound diets and discovered that animals on fad diets lost weight sooner, but those on well-balanced diets eventually lost as much weight and more body fat (instead of muscle tissue). After a fad diet, you may weigh less – but you have a higher percentage of body fat.

A too-rich diet raises your setpoint. Bet you're not surprised. When laboratory animals are fed food that's fatty and sugary, they eat more of it. Rats, which don't usually become fat, *will* gain weight on what's called a cafeteria diet – that's peanut butter, sandwich cookies, fruit punches, and all the other things that taste good and are bad for you. Foods in that category are low in nutritional value, so Nature made sure that animals would get all the nutrition necessary from 'junk food' by overeating it on the rare occasions when they'd come across it. When Nature set this up, of course, she didn't know bags full of sugared popcorn and gallons of ice cream loaded with butterfat would one day be as close as the nearest supermarket.

Eating frequently helps you stay fit. There is some evidence that when you eat only one big meal a day, you store more food than if you eat several times a day; scientists don't know why this is true, but your fat-storing pathways seem to operate better when you eat once daily. Also, the very act of eating seems to burn off calories, which is why sometimes eating regularly is more effective than fasting. The name for this phenomenon is *diet-induced thermogenesis*.

What Is Thermogenesis?

Your body uses food in three ways. Some of it is used to keep your system going – to do everything from breathing to moving. Some food goes into storage. And some of it is lost as heat. That process is called thermogenesis. (Think of the heat generated by almost every working machine you can think of.) One example of thermogenesis is heat given off from eating. Think of the advice to starve a fever – the act of eating raises the amount of heat produced by your body, which is not desirable when your temperature is already elevated. Shivering is another kind of thermogenesis; it happens when your body tries to make you warmer.

If you're too fat, you want to increase thermogenesis so that your body loses more food as heat and stores less food as fat. There are two influences on body thermogenesis. One is the brown fat I mentioned earlier, but no one knows how to increase the amount of brown fat yet. The other influence is skeletal muscle (as opposed to organ muscle, like the heart). We do know how to do something about skeletal muscle – you can build it up, and thus build up the thermogenetic effect, through exercise.

Exercise Is as Important as Diet

Exercise has several important roles. One, it increases the amount of skeletal muscle. A person whose body has a higher percentage of lean muscle loses more calories thermogenetically, as heat. Besides, increasing your skeletal muscle as you diet will prevent that gaunt look that makes everyone tell you you look 'too thin' while they tell Bo Derek she's just right. Dieters who look gaunt have simply lost too much muscle. (Besides, when you don't use your muscle, part of that muscle fibre just won't grow back. If muscles are out of shape, they lose the 'girdle' effect on your layers of fat tissue.)

The idea is to replace fat with muscle. My mother warned me that if I exercised my fat would turn into muscle. Well, now I have something to tell you, Mother. Fat has about as much chance of turning into muscle as Kermit does of turning into a prince. Your muscle looks like a nicely marbled steak: your goal is to burn up the fat and retain the muscle. In fact, all you can do is burn the fat: you can't change it into muscle.

Interestingly, since muscle weighs more than fat, as you build up muscle, you may weigh a bit more on the scale, but your clothes will be getting looser. (Reducing your calories while you exercise will, of course, result in a net weight loss.)

The other role of exercise is to increase your metabolic rate. You used to be told that such and such exercise used up so many calories. Actually, it has a much more important effect. Now scientists have discovered that exercise can speed up your metabolic rate for as long as twenty-four hours. Long after the exercise is over, your body is burning up calories more quickly while you're moving normally and even as you sleep.

As a bonus, scientists also think that exercise within an hour or so after a meal speeds up diet-induced thermogenesis.

The right kind of exercise is steady and calls for a lot of endurance. Since you're not trying to build up muscle, but rather to burn off fat, you need what's called an 'aerobic exercise'. Of them all, for reasons soon explained, we've chosen walking.

Finally, you need to change some of your habits. Your regulatory system may be off. Researchers speculate that is why fat people so often depend on outside clues (seeing that the clock reads noon) rather than inner ones (feeling their stomachs growling) to move them to eat.

In order to lose weight, you must replace some of these clues with new ones. If passing the bakery is enough to trigger you to buy an éclair, then you must avoid passing the bakery. You must consciously substitute new, helpful habits for old, harmful ones. Dr Joel indicated some ways to change my behaviour, and I discovered some of my own. You can read them in the pages that follow.

Now That You Understand the Reasons Behind the Help Yourself Plan, Here Is a Brief Description

THE EIGHT–STEP HELP YOURSELF DIET PLAN

Step	How Long	Daily Diet	Exercise
1	ONE WEEK	1000 calories (Menus provided)	20 minutes moderate walking, 5 times weekly
2	ONE WEEK or until within four pounds of goal	1000 calories (Menus provided)	30 minutes moderate walking, 5 times weekly
3	UNTIL WITHIN FOUR POUNDS OF GOAL	1000 calories (Self-selection)	60 minutes including warm-up, cool down, 30 minutes of brisk walking, 5 times weekly
4	UNTIL WITHIN TWO POUNDS OF GOAL	1200 calories (Self-selection)	Continue Step 3
5	UNTIL AT GOAL	1400 calories (Self-selection)	Continue Step 3
6	UNTIL ONE POUND *BELOW* GOAL	1600 calories (Self-selection)	Continue Step 3

Step	How Long	Daily Diet	Exercise
7	UNTIL TWO POUNDS *BELOW* GOAL	1800 calories (Self-selection)	Continue Step 3
8*	UNTIL YOU HAVE GAINED 1–2 POUNDS	2000 calories or more (Self-selection)	Continue Step 3

If, for any reason, you gain, drop your calorie intake 400 calories daily until you are back to goal weight. Never return to the 800- or 1000-calorie level.

Note:
• A diet diary *must* be kept throughout. See Part Three: Second Helpings (page 250) for sample.
• Drink six to eight glasses of water or enough to pass at least a quart of urine daily.
• Ask your doctor to recommend a multivitamin to take daily. Take it along with the meal in which you have the most fat, since certain vitamins are only absorbed in the presence of fat.
• If you feel tired or don't feel yourself, check with your doctor.

Goal weight may be determined from the latest Metropolitan Life Insurance Company height and weight chart, published December 1982. Most charts used in Britain are based on it, so any chart from a reputable source, such as an established diet food manufacturer, will do. Since you will be more muscular than you used to be (and muscle,

*In Step 8, add calories in 200-calorie increments weekly until you have gained 1–2 pounds. Determine your calorie needs by picking a mid-point between the calorie intake on which you were losing and the calorie intake on which you are now gaining. You may find you are comfortable at a goal weight higher than originally anticipated since your body is in better shape. *You are now stabilized at your goal weight.* You must continue to exercise.

as you know, weighs more than fat), you might find yourself revising your personal goal weight upwards as you stay on the programme. You may look and feel better at a higher weight than you had originally planned.

A Two-Week Shopping List for the 1000-Calorie Diet

To make it easy for you to start your diet, I've made up a shopping list. It includes everything you'll need over the first two weeks on your diet. In order to vary the menu, I've included some items you can't buy in small enough quantities, so you may have extra of some items. Freeze it or *give it away* if you must.

Meat and Fish	*Week 1*	*Week 2*
Tuna, canned, in brine	1 can (6½ oz/185 g)	1 can (6½ oz/185 g)
Prawns, canned		1 can (7 oz/198 g)
Chicken, skinned and boned breast	11 oz/300 g	8 oz/225 g
Sirloin steak, lean	5 oz/150 g	6½ oz/185 g
Hamburger, lean		4 oz/100 g
Pork chop, boned and trimmed or fillet	5 oz/150 g	5 oz/150 g
Cod or mullet or	7 oz/200 g	
Scallops	6 oz/175 g	
Plaice or sole, fillet	6 oz/175 g	12 oz/340 g
Rabbit or guinea fowl	16 oz/450 g	
Prawns, fresh, in shell	8 oz/225 g	
Lean gammon rashers	2 oz/50 g	1 oz/25 g
Lamb chops or cutlets		2 5-oz/150-g chops
Dairy Products		
Skim milk	2 pints	1 pint
Eggs	3	4

	Week 1	Week 2
Vanilla or lemon low-fat yogurt	8 oz/225 g	8 oz/225 g
Plain low-fat yogurt	8 oz/225 g	12 oz/340 g
Parmesan cheese	small carton (1½ oz/ 42.5 g)	
Butter or margarine	4 oz/100 g	

Starches

	Week 1	Week 2
Whole grain breakfast cereal (choose from calorie counter, p. 133)	1 box	
Rolled oats	1 box	
Whole wheat bread, thinly sliced	7 slices	12 slices
Whole wheat melba toast	1 box	
Rice, white, quick cooking	1 box	
Egg noodles	1 box	
Popcorn	1 packet, unpopped	
Waffles, frozen jumbo (Downyflake or Aunt Jemima)	2 waffles	2 waffles

Fruit and Vegetables – Fresh

	Week 1	Week 2
Medium bananas (6"/15 cm)	3	1
Strawberries	approx. 12 oz/340 g	approx. 9 oz/250 g
Medium peaches (if not in season, substitute tangerine, ½ pear, or 6 oz/175 g chunk unsweetened pineapple in its own juice)	3	4
Cantaloupe melon (if not in season, substitute ½ grapefruit for each ¼ melon)	1	1

	Week 1	*Week 2*
Medium apples (2¼"/5.5 cm diameter)	5	6
Medium oranges	3	2
Grapefruit		1
Green pepper	1	1
Tomatoes, medium	3	3
Green beans	3 oz/75 g	5½ oz/165 g
Beetroot (3½ oz/85 g each)	2	
Courgette (1 medium, about 6 oz/175 g)		1
Celery	2 stalks	2 stalks
Broccoli	4 medium spears	8 medium spears
Swede, 1 small	½	½
Carrots, medium	5	3
Cucumber	1	
Asparagus (frozen if necessary)	10 spears	
Mushrooms	6 oz/175 g	6 oz/175 g
Lettuce, small head	1	1
Baking potato, approx. 5½ oz/ 160 g	2	1
Parsnips		1 lb/450 g
Parsley (optional)	1 small bunch	
Chives (optional)	1 bunch	
Garlic	1 clove	

Other

Raisins	small package	
Unsweetened apple sauce	1 8-oz/225-g jar	
Frozen orange juice concentrate	1 small can	
Lemon juice	1 squeeze bottle	

	Week 1	*Week 2*
Prepared mustard (optional)	1 small jar	
Vegetable oil	1 bottle	
Low-calorie salad dressing (1T.* = 20 calories)	1 bottle	
Low-calorie mayonnaise	1 jar	
Dry mustard		
Paprika		
Ginger		
Cinnamon		
Nutmeg		

FOURTEEN DAYS OF 1000-CALORIE† MENUS

DAY 1

Breakfast

¾ oz/20 g unsweetened whole grain breakfast cereal	70
4 fl oz/120 ml skim milk	45
½ medium banana	45
	160

Lunch

Sandwich made with:

2 thin slices whole wheat bread	80
½ 6½-oz/185-g can tuna in brine	110

*T. = tablespoon/15 ml spoon.

†A brief calorie counter is found in Part Three: Second Helpings, page 246. Calories have been rounded off to the nearest whole number. You'll see that calories don't come out to exactly 1000 every day – the total on some days will be slightly under and on others slightly over.

½ T. low-calorie mayonnaise	20
½ tomato	15
lettuce leaf	0
¼ cantaloupe melon	35
4 fl oz/120 ml skim milk	45
	305

Dinner

5 oz/150 g (raw weight) lean sirloin steak, grilled	300
1 potato, baked	90
with 1 tsp.* margarine or butter	35
2 oz/50 g mushroom, cooked	15
5 asparagus spears, steamed	20
2 medium carrots, steamed	40
	500

Snack

1 medium apple	80
	1040

Helpful Hints for Day 1

- Slice the remaining half of banana from this morning's breakfast, wrap tightly in an airtight bag, then freeze. Tomorrow evening mix it with the vanilla yogurt and strawberries for a nice ice-cream type dessert.
- If you must use a leftover can of tuna in oil, be sure you rinse it under cold running water and pat dry with paper towels before eating.
- Cooked meat shrinks. I've given you specific raw weights to buy throughout the fourteen days, but you might want to know the rules of thumb for future use. Beef: expect 1 oz/25 g shrinkage for every 4 oz/100 g purchased. Chicken: 6 oz/175 g with bones will yield 3 oz/75 g of cooked meat. Fish: 10 oz/275 g will give you 5 oz/150 g fillet.

* tsp. = teaspoon/5 ml spoon.

- For mushrooms in a light gravy: wash just before you use them by rinsing briefly in cool water, then blot with a damp paper towel. Put in a frying pan with enough water to cover them half-way, add paprika and pepper, and simmer briefly until mushrooms are soft.

Comments from Mary Ellen on Day 1

- At first the portions may look very small to you. They did to me. I had never dealt with spoonful measurements, for instance. Let me assure you that once the food is on your plate, you'll be surprised. There's a lot there.
- I felt full on 1000 calories because I was used to no breakfast, a light lunch, and then a six-hour dinner. When's the last time you ate three meals a day?
- If you experience true hunger, don't snack. Drink a couple of glasses of water or go for a walk. It'll soon disappear.
- And finally, congratulations on your good start at Helping Yourself. Keep going.

DAY 2

Breakfast

1 whole egg, poached	75
1 thin slice whole wheat bread	40
¼ cantaloupe melon	35
	150

Lunch

MIX TOGETHER:

4 oz/100 g plain yogurt	70
½ cucumber, diced	10
1 medium tomato	30
1 stalk celery, diced	10
½ green pepper, chopped	10
	105

3 slices whole wheat melba toast	45
1 medium peach	40
	215

Dinner

6 oz/175 g skinned and boned breast of chicken, baked	300
4 medium spears fresh broccoli	40
with 1 tsp. margarine or butter and	35
1 tsp. Parmesan cheese	10
3 oz/75 g cooked rice	80
with 1 tsp. margarine or butter and	35
½ tsp. chopped parsley	0
	500

Snack

½ medium banana, sliced	45
3 oz/75 g sliced strawberries	25
mixed with 2 oz/50 g vanilla yogurt	50
	120
	985

Helpful Hints for Day 2

- The best-tasting cantaloupe melons should have no greenish cast to the skin. A ripe one will have a pleasant smell and will yield to slight finger pressure at the blossom end – the end opposite the stem.
- Have a cucumber to peel and can't find your potato peeler? Use a spatula-type cheese slicer to get the job done quickly.
- Cook tonight's chicken plus an additional 4 oz/100 g to use for lunch tomorrow and Day 5.
- Don't buy chicken with brownish areas: it's been in the supermarket fridge too long or been stored improperly.

Forget it, also, if the skin looks dry, purplish, bruised or scaly.
- Keep parsley fresh and crisp by storing in a wide-mouth jar with a tight lid.
- Add artificial sweetener to the yogurt if you need a sweeter treat. Try different brands of yogurt, since they vary in consistency and tartness; but be sure to check the label for the calorie count.

DAY 3

Breakfast
¾ oz/20 g unsweetened whole grain breakfast cereal	70
4 fl oz/120 ml skim milk	45
¼ cantaloupe melon	35
	150

Lunch
Salad made with:
diced cooked chicken (2 oz/50 g raw)	100
1 medium apple, diced	80
1 stalk celery, diced	10
1 T. low-calorie mayonnaise	40
¼ cucumber	5
served on lettuce leaves	0
2 slices whole wheat melba toast	30
	265

Dinner
6 oz/175 g (raw weight) plaice or sole, baked or grilled with a squeeze of lemon juice	150
½ tomato, baked or grilled	15
with 1 T. Parmesan cheese	25

107

8 oz/225 g swede, baked	80
with 1 tsp. margarine or butter	35
1½ oz/35 g green beans	25
with 1 tsp. butter or margarine	35
3 oz/75 g strawberries, sliced, with	25
½ medium banana, sliced	45
	435

Snack

popcorn, 1 oz/25 g popped with ½ T. oil	
or 1½ oz/35 g popped without oil	160
	950

Helpful Hints for Day 3

- Line the bottom of your salad crisper with paper towels to keep lettuce fresh and crisp longer. The paper towels absorb all the excess moisture.
- Strawberries can be kept firm for several days if you store them in a colander in the refrigerator, which allows the cold air to circulate around them. Don't hull them until they have been washed or they will absorb too much water and become mushy.
- Cooking a perfect fish is easy, if you remember this ten-minute rule – whether you're grilling, baking, simmering, poaching or steaming fresh (not frozen) fish. A 1 inch/2.5 cm thick piece takes ten minutes to cook. Add two minutes' cooking time for every ¼ inch/5 mm above 1 inch/2.5 cm, and subtract two minutes for every ¼ inch/5 mm below. Plaice, at about ¼ inch/5 mm, will cook in 3–4 minutes, 1¼ inch/3 cm salmon in 12–13.
- Slice tomatoes vertically and the slices stay firm while baking.
- Lower-calorie popcorn: cover the pan bottom with salt instead of oil or butter. Heat the salt, then add the popcorn.

DAY 4

Breakfast

¾ oz/20 g unsweetened whole grain breakfast cereal	70
4 fl oz/120 ml skim milk	45
3 oz/75 g strawberries	25
	140

Lunch

Sandwich made with:

1 thin slice whole wheat bread	40
½ 6½-oz/185-g can tuna in brine	110
½ T. low-calorie mayonnaise	20
1 T. Parmesan cheese (sprinkle on top and place sandwich under grill or in microwave oven briefly)	25
1 medium apple	80
	275

Dinner

8 oz/225 g prawns (raw), peeled and deveined	200
(sauté in ½ T. vegetable oil with	50
1 clove minced garlic)	0
3 oz/75 g cooked rice	80

Salad made with:

½ small head lettuce	25
½ carrot, chopped	10
½ tomato, chopped	15
2 tsp. Parmesan cheese	15
1 T. low-calorie salad dressing	20
asparagus, 5 spears, steamed	20
	435

Snack

4 oz/100 g plain yogurt with	70
1 sliced fresh peach	40
	110
	960

Helpful Hints for Day 4

- After shelling and deveining prawns, put them in a bowl and wash gently under cold, running water for half a minute. Next, rinse them in a colander under briskly running cold water for about three minutes. When cooked, they will almost crunch.
- Remove the tops of carrots before storing in the refrigerator. Tops drain the carrots of moisture, making them limp and dry.
- Asparagus, like broad beans, sweetcorn, and spinach, loses moisture fast. It should be refrigerated the moment you come home from the market.

DAY 5

Breakfast

1 thin slice whole wheat toast	40
1 whole egg, scrambled in non-stick pan	75
1 medium orange	80
	195

Lunch

Sandwich made with:

1 thin slice whole wheat bread	40
1 T. low-calorie mayonnaise	40

sliced chicken without skin	
(2 oz/50 g raw weight)	100
lettuce leaf	0
1 medium apple	80
	260

Dinner

7 oz/200 g cod or mullet *or* 6 oz/175 g	
scallops, grilled with lemon and paprika	190
1½ oz/35 g raw egg noodles, steamed	100
2 beetroot, steamed	30
1 tsp. margarine or butter	35
1 sliced fresh peach	40
	395

Snack

2 slices melba toast with	30
1 tsp. margarine or butter, sprinkled with cinnamon	35
4 oz/100 g vanilla yogurt	100
	165
	1015

Helpful Hints for Day 5
- The larger apples have more than 80 calories; besides, small and medium fruits are generally tastier than large ones.
- Apples should be smooth, firm to the touch and free of bruises. Avoid red apples that are greenish; pass by Golden Delicious apples that are very large and deeply yellow. Both are a sign of ageing and mealiness.
- For silky-smooth scrambled eggs, start with a cool non-stick pan and cook eggs very slowly.
- Put young beetroot tops in the freezer for eventual use. Boil gently and chop like spinach.

DAY 6

Breakfast

1 oz/25 g rolled oats	100
with 1 medium apple, chopped	80
and cinnamon to taste	0
4 fl oz/120 ml skim milk	45
	225

Lunch

Salad made with:

½ small head lettuce	25
½ green pepper, chopped	10
½ carrot, sliced	10
2 oz/50 g mushrooms, sliced	15
½ tomato, chopped	15
¼ cucumber, chopped	5
1 hard-boiled egg, chopped	75
1 T. low-calorie salad dressing	20
3 slices whole wheat melba toast	45
1 medium banana	90
	310

Dinner

5 oz/150 g (raw weight) pork chop, grilled	300
1 medium potato, baked, with 1 tsp.	90
margarine or butter	35
1½ oz/35 g green beans, steamed, with a	
squeeze of lemon juice	25
	450

Snack

1 medium orange	80
	——
	1065

Helpful Hints for Day 6

- Store apples alone. Apples tend to give off a gas that can make carrots bitter.
- You can substitute the Special Vinaigrette (see page 225) for low-calorie salad dressing.
- There's more to making hard-boiled eggs than you might think. Place eggs in a pan, cover with cold water, and pour in some vinegar or salt. The vinegar keeps the egg from oozing out if the shell cracks while cooking. Bring to a boil and remove from heat. Set in covered pan for twenty minutes. Drain off hot water. Now, shake the pan back and forth, causing the eggs to crack against the side. Cool with cold water and peel.
- Use an egg slicer to slice mushrooms uniformly and easily.
- Bumps on green beans mean they are tough, so there is more waste. Select young, small ones.
- Rough, pitted skin may indicate that an orange is dry, so choose oranges with smooth, thin skin.

DAY 7

Brunch

2 medium waffles with	170
4 oz/100 g unsweetened apple sauce	50
2 oz/50 g lean gammon rashers	90
¼ cantaloupe melon	40
	——
	350

Dinner

5 oz/150 g boned rabbit meat	250
(baste with 2 tsp. frozen orange juice	10
concentrate mixed with 1 tsp. water	0
and a pinch of ground ginger if desired)	0
3 oz/75 g cooked rice with	80
½ tsp. margarine or butter	20
½ tsp. chopped parsley	0
2 oz/50 g sliced mushrooms	15
2 carrots, steamed with	40
1 tsp. margarine or butter	35
1 medium orange, sliced	80
	530

Snack

2 oz/50 g vanilla yogurt	50
½ medium banana, sliced	45
3 oz/75 g sliced strawberries	25
	120
	1000

Helpful Hints for Day 7
- Mix cinnamon, nutmeg, ginger, and cloves to taste if you want a spicier apple sauce; or use ground mixed spice.
- To store unused frozen orange juice concentrate, remove needed concentrate without thawing all the juice by running hot water over the outside of the can until concentrate is softened just enough to use. Then cover the top surface with plastic wrap and secure the top of can with a rubber band. Replace can in the freezer.
- Mushrooms won't get slimy if you refrigerate them in a brown paper bag. Paper allows the mushrooms

to 'breathe' while keeping in the humidity that keeps them fresh.
- Or, store mushrooms, already sliced, in your freezer.

DAY 8

Breakfast

1 thin slice whole wheat toast	40
1 tsp. margarine or butter	35
1 whole egg, scrambled with	75
1 T. skim milk	10
½ grapefruit	40
	200

Lunch

Sandwich made with:

1 thin slice whole wheat bread	40
3½ oz/85 g canned prawns, drained	115
1 T. low-calorie mayonnaise	40
lettuce leaf	0
1 medium peach	40
	235

Dinner

5 oz/150 g (raw weight) sirloin steak, grilled	300
2 oz/50 g mushrooms, cooked	15
3 oz/75 g egg noodles, boiled, with	100
½ tsp. margarine or butter and	20
½ tsp. chopped parsley	0
2 carrots, steamed	40
	475

Snack

4 oz/100 g plain yogurt with	70
2 tsp. frozen orange juice concentrate	10
½ medium banana, sliced	45

	125

	1035

Helpful Hints for Day 8
- To keep the other half grapefruit fresh, put it cut side down in a small bowl and refrigerate.
- Buy grapefruit that's heavy for its size (test in your palm) and thin-skinned. Pink looks pretty but tastes exactly like yellow and costs more.
- Store leftover canned prawns in a tightly covered refrigerator dish or plastic bag, not in the can.
- Grill the remaining 1½ oz/35 g steak for lunch Day 9.
- When you buy carrots, buy them with tops off. They lose moisture through those pretty green leaves.

DAY 9

Breakfast

1 oz/25 g rolled oats with	100
1 T. raisins, cinnamon and nutmeg	30
4 fl oz/120 ml skim milk	45
¼ cantaloupe melon	40

	215

Lunch
Sandwich made with:

1 thin slice whole wheat bread	40
1½ oz/35 g (raw weight) sliced cooked sirloin steak	90

½ small tomato, sliced	15
1 tsp. mustard	5
lettuce leaf	0
1 medium apple	80
	230

Dinner

6 oz/150 g sole or plaice, grilled or baked	150
8 oz/225 g swede, baked,	80
topped with 1 tsp. margarine	
or butter	35
pinch of cinnamon	0
Salad made with:	
½ small head lettuce	25
½ carrot, chopped	20
2 oz/50 g mushrooms, sliced	15
1 T. low-calorie salad dressing	20
1 potato, baked	90
1 medium peach	40
	475

Snack

1 medium orange	80
	1000

Helpful Hints for Day 9
- Take the lumps out of cooked cereal by whipping with a wire whisk.
- Store raisins in a cool, dry place until you open the package, then put them in a plastic bag and store in the refrigerator.
- When selecting carrots, bear in mind that young, slender ones are usually sweeter. Thick carrots, deeper in colour, are older and would be better for stews and soups.

● If tiny flies are buzzing around peaches (or cherries or plums) don't buy them. It means the fruit is over-ripe. Don't buy when green, either. Peaches won't ripen at home.

DAY 10

Breakfast

2 slices whole wheat toast	80
4 oz/100 g plain yogurt with	70
3 oz/75 g strawberries	25
1 tsp. orange juice concentrate	10
	185

Lunch

Salad made with:

½ small head lettuce	25
½ 6½-oz/185-g can tuna in brine	110
½ carrot, chopped	20
1 stalk celery, chopped	10
1 T. low-calorie salad dressing	20
1 medium apple	80
	265

Dinner

6 oz/175 g (raw weight) boneless, skinless chicken breast, baked	300
1 courgette (approx. 6 oz/175 g), steamed,	20
topped with 1 tsp. Parmesan cheese	10
3 oz/75 g cooked rice with	80
1 tsp. margarine or butter	35
	445

Snack

2 oz/50 g vanilla yogurt	50
1 fresh peach, sliced	40
	90
	985

Helpful Hints for Day 10

- An easy way to slice or chop carrots is to put the whole carrot inside the curve of a celery stalk. The carrot doesn't roll around – and you'll have both vegetables sliced or chopped at one time.
- Bake an additional 2 oz/50 g (raw weight) of chicken to be used for lunch on Day 11.
- Realize that by cooking your own chicken, you are saving not only calories but also money. Prepared chicken costs four times as much as fresh.
- An easy way to peel peaches: dip the fruit into boiling water for fifteen seconds, then dip into cold water (to prevent cooking). The skin will slide right off.

DAY 11

Breakfast

¾ oz/20 g whole grain breakfast cereal	70
4 fl oz/120 ml skim milk	45
3 oz/75 g strawberries	25
	140

Lunch

Sandwich made with:

2 thin slices whole wheat bread	80

119

sliced chicken without skin	
(2 oz/50 g raw weight)	100
½ tomato, sliced	15
1 T. low-calorie mayonnaise	40
lettuce leaf	0
1 medium apple	80
	315

Dinner

4 oz/100 g lean hamburger, grilled	240
6 T. unsweetened apple sauce	35
1 small sweet potato or yam, baked with	140
1 tsp. margarine or butter	35
2 oz/50 g steamed green beans, with	30
1 tsp. margarine or butter	35
	515

Snack

1 medium orange	80
	1050

Helpful Hints for Day 11

- The tip of your potato peeler is great for removing the stems from strawberries. Just insert it underneath the stem cap, hold the cap with your thumb and lift off quickly and easily.
- Buy tomatoes with the stem attached. The tiny stem helps keep in moisture.
- Use a melon baller to core an apple half quickly and easily.
- You can cut the baking time by as much as half if you place potatoes on the oven rack and then place an iron pot over them.

DAY 12

Breakfast

1 waffle	85
1 tsp. margarine or butter	35
4 oz/100 g vanilla yogurt	100
½ medium banana	45
	225

Lunch

Sandwich made with:

1 thin slice whole wheat bread	40
½ 6½-oz/185-g can prawns, drained	115
1 stalk celery, diced	10
1 T. low-calorie mayonnaise	40
pinch of dry mustard	0
3 oz/75 g sliced strawberries	25
	230

Dinner

2 5-oz/150-g (raw weight) grilled lamb chops (eat *lean* meat only)	250
3 oz/75 g rice, steamed, with	80
1 tsp. margarine or butter	35
1 small tomato, sliced, with	30
1 T. low-calorie salad dressing	20
4 spears broccoli	20
	435

Snack

4 oz/100 g plain yogurt with	70
2 tsp. frozen orange juice concentrate	10
1 medium peach, sliced	40
	120
	1005

Help Yourself: the Programme

Helpful Hints for Day 12

- Canned prawns lose their 'canned' taste if you soak them for fifteen minutes in two tablespoons of vinegar and a teaspoon of sherry.
- They may look pretty, but skip the giant strawberries. Sweetest are medium-sized, no larger than a 10p piece.
- Green tomatoes ripen in a cool, dark corner.

DAY 13

Breakfast

1 thin slice whole wheat bread	40
with 1 tsp. margarine or butter	35
1 egg, poached	75
1 medium apple	80
	230

Lunch

1 small tomato, cut in wedges	30
Salad made of:	
½ 6½-oz/185-g can tuna in brine	110
½ green pepper, diced	10
1 T. low-calorie mayonnaise	40
pinch of dry mustard	0
pinch of paprika	0
2 slices whole wheat melba toast	30
1 medium peach or ½ eating pear	40
	260

Dinner

6 oz/150 g (raw weight) plaice or sole, baked or grilled	150

3 oz/75 g green beans with	50
1 tsp. margarine or butter	35
8 oz/225 g parsnips baked with	140
1 tsp. butter or margarine	35
½ cantaloupe melon	35
	415

Snack

1 medium apple	80
	985

Helpful Hints for Day 13
- If poached eggs can't be served immediately, put them in cool water and when you're ready to serve, reheat them gently in hot, salted water.
- Paprika will keep its colour and flavour longer if it is stored in the refrigerator.

DAY 14

Brunch

Omelette made with:	
1 whole egg and 1 egg white	90
1 T. Parmesan cheese	25
½ green pepper, chopped	10
2 oz/50 g mushrooms, sliced	15
1 oz/25 g lean gammon rashers, diced	45
2 slices whole wheat toast	80
with 2 T. unsweetened apple sauce and cinnamon	15
½ grapefruit	40
	320

Dinner

5 oz/150 g (raw weight) pork chop, grilled	300
4 spears broccoli, steamed	40
with 1 tsp. butter or margarine	35
squeeze of lemon juice	0
3 oz/75 g egg noodles, boiled, with	100
½ tsp. margarine or butter	35
½ tsp. chives	0
½ cantaloupe melon with	70
2 oz/50 g vanilla yogurt	50
	——
	630

Snack

1 medium apple	80
	——
	1030

Helpful Hints for Day 14

- You may want to make your own apple sauce for the diet. After peeling two apples, use a hand grater to slice them into a pot containing 4 fl oz/120 ml water. Cover and simmer until the apples are tender. Then, using a wire whisk, blend the apples to the correct consistency.
- Thick broccoli stems can be cooked in the same length of time as the florets if you make 'X' incisions from top to bottom along the stem. Cook the dark green leaves, too: they are extremely nutritious.

11. Now That You're Ready to Choose Your Own Menus . . .

I know that you're nervous. You're more comfortable with structure, but you've got to learn how to eat like a normal person, and you might as well start now. So you're going to find out how to construct your own diet, which, when you think about it, makes the most sense. If *you* select it, you'll be less likely to rebel against it.

The basic system that follows was developed by many professional health organizations such as the American Dietetic Association. It's especially designed to be used as a life-long plan, and our nutritionist modified it to co-ordinate with your exercise programme and take advantage of the latest information on the topic of obesity.

The best part about it is that you'll be eating normal – not diet – foods, which is appropriate if you're going to live the rest of your life like a normal, fit person. This also makes it easy to eat out and cook at home, but it does require a little planning ahead.

Remember: as you lose weight, you must add calories in order to prevent your metabolism from slowing down. You may want some advice as to how you do this. Obviously, you don't just add a scoop of ice cream for each 200-calorie increase you're allowed. For guidance, you can use the chart on page 128. (Remember also, if you gain a pound or two, cut back to 400 calories until you're at goal. The system that follows can be adapted for this purpose, too.)

Say you're planning a 1200-calorie day. As you read down the column, you see you can have 1 milk, 1 fruit, 1 bread, 2 meat, and 1 fat serving for breakfast, and so on for lunch. These servings come from the lists of Food Groups that follow. In the sample below, I'm going to list calories, but there's actually an easy trick to this. If you follow the food groups, the calories, proteins, carbohydrates, fat, vitamins, and minerals will *automatically* equal up to a balanced diet.

SAMPLE 1200-CALORIE DIET

Food Group/Serving	Menu Item	Calorie Count
Breakfast		
1 Milk + 1 Fat	8 oz/225 g low-fat yogurt	125
1 Fruit	5 oz/150 g strawberries	40
1 Starch	½ muffin	70
2 Meat (includes 1 Fat)	2 oz/50 g skim mozzarella	140
Misc./unlimited	Black coffee	0
		350
Lunch		
1 Free Vegetable	Lettuce	0
2 Meat (low fat)	2 oz/50 g boiled prawns	110
1 Fat	2 tsp. low-calorie mayonnaise	45
2 Starch	2 slices whole wheat bread	140
1 Fruit	2 medium plums	40
Misc./unlimited	Slimline American Ginger Ale (restrict to 2 daily)	0
		335
Dinner		
1 Vegetable	3 oz/75 g spinach and mushroom salad	25

Food Group/Serving	Menu Item	Calorie Count
2 Fat	2 T. oil	90
Free	Vinegar	0
2 Low-fat Meat	Grilled chicken	110
2 Starch	6 oz/175 g baked or boiled potato	140
1 Fruit	½ grapefruit	40
		405

Snack		
1 Milk	4 fl oz/120 ml skim milk	80
1 Fruit	1 peach	40
		120

As you get familiar with the lists of Food Groups that follow, you'll soon know which foods are lowest in fat, which are similar in nutritional content, and which can be eaten in any amounts. All of the following Food Group lists contain foods that are approximately equal in protein, carbohydrate, and fat – plus vitamins and minerals.

If you are going out for a special dinner, or if you plan to combine two meals such as brunch, you can swap foods from two meals. As a rule, though, you are advised to eat three standard meals plus a fourth light meal such as milk and fruit.

What the Food Groups Consist Of
What follows is some of my favourite reading matter – lists of foods. Since the lists are meant to help guide you until you're living like a normal person, many non-diet foods do appear. Of course, it would be impossible to list every food you're likely to eat, but these lists should help guide your selection until you're stabilized at your goal weight.

Normal, fit people don't consult charts when they eat, and

neither will you eventually. I hope by the time you feel comfortable without instructions, you will have absorbed the basic principles of sound eating and they'll be second nature.

One final comment about the lists that follow: don't obsess. The calorie counts are meant to be guidelines. If you notice a ten-calorie discrepancy between one calorie count and another, don't be concerned. I can assure you that such a discrepancy won't make a significant difference in your weight loss.

FOOD GROUPS ACCORDING TO CALORIC INTAKE

Calories	1000	1200	1400	1600	1800	2000
Food Group						
Breakfast						
Milk	1	1	1	1	1	1
Fruit	1	1	1	1	1	1
Starch	1	1	2	3	3	3
Meat*	2	2	2	2	2	2
Fat	1	1	1	1	2	2
Lunch						
Free veg.	any	any	any	any	any	any
Fruit	1	1	2	2	3	3
Starch	2	2	2	2	3	3
Meat*	2	2	2	3	3	3
Fat	1	1	2	2	2	3
Dinner						
Milk	0	0	0	0	0	1
Vegetable	1	1	1	1	2	2

*Use low-fat meat at least two out of three times daily. This group is lowest in cholesterol as well as fat and calories.

Calories	1000	1200	1400	1600	1800	2000
Food Group						
Fruit	1	1	2	2	2	2
Starch	1	2	2	2	3	3
Meat*	2	2	2	3	3	3
Fat	1	2	2	2	2	3
Snack						
Milk	0	1	1	1	1	1
Fruit	1	1	1	1	1	1
Summary						
Milk	1	2	2	2	2	3
Fruit	4	4	6	6	6	6
Starch	4	5	6	7	9	9
Meat	6	6	6	8	8	8
Vegetable	2	2	2	2	3	3
Fat	3	4	4	5	6	8

Milk Group

Per serving: 12 grams of carbohydrate, 8 grams of protein, a trace of fat, and 80 calories. Milk products are a major source of calcium, a good source of phosphorus, protein, some B vitamins, vitamins A and D, and some magnesium.

NON-FAT
skim milk	8 fl oz/225 ml
canned evaporated skim milk	4 fl oz/120 ml
powdered non-fat dry milk (before adding liquid)	1 oz/25 g
plain yogurt made from skim milk	8 fl oz/225 ml

*Use low-fat meat at least two out of three times daily. This group is lowest in cholesterol as well as fat and calories.

M.E.–E

LOW FAT*

low-fat milk, 98 per cent fat free	8 fl oz/225 ml
low-fat buttermilk	8 fl oz/225 ml
plain yogurt made from low-fat milk	8 fl oz/225 ml

FULL FAT†

whole milk	4 fl oz/120 ml
goat's milk	4 fl oz/120 ml
canned evaporated whole milk	2 fl oz/60 ml
powdered dry milk (before adding liquid)	3 T.
plain yogurt made from whole milk	4 fl oz/120 ml

Fruit Group

Per serving: 10 grams of carbohydrate and 40 calories. Fruits contain a variety of vitamins and minerals, and are a good source of fibre. Citrus fruits are the best source of vitamin C.

BERRY FRUITS

blackberries	6 oz/175 g
loganberries	6 oz/175 g
mulberries	4 oz/100 g
cranberries	8 oz/225 g
raspberries	5 oz/150 g
strawberries	5 oz/150 g

CITRUS FRUITS

grapefruit	½
orange	½ small
tangerine, satsuma, clementine	1 medium

* For each serving you select from this group, omit 1 FAT serving from your day's total.

† For each serving you select from this group, omit 2 FAT servings from your day's total.

DRIED FRUITS
  apricots   4 halves
  dates   2 medium
  figs   1 medium
  peaches   2 halves
  pears   2 halves
  prunes   2 medium
  raisins, sultanas   2 tsp.

FRUIT JUICES
  apple   ⅛ pint/75 ml
  cranberry   2 fl oz/60 ml
  grape   2 fl oz/60 ml
  grapefruit   4 fl oz/120 ml
  orange   4 fl oz/120 ml
  papaya   ⅛ pint/75 ml
  pineapple   ⅛ pint/75 ml
  prune   2 fl oz/60 ml

MELONS
  cantaloupe   ¼
  honeydew   ⅛
  watermelon   approx. ½
                                      centre slice,
                                      diced

OTHER FRUITS
  apple   ½ small
  apple sauce   4 oz/100 g
  apricots   2 medium
  banana   ½ small
  cherries   10 large
  grapes   12
  kiwi fruit   1 medium
  mango   ½ small
  nectarine   1 small
  pawpaw   1 large

papaya	⅓ medium *or* ½ small
peach	1 medium
pear	1 medium
persimmon	1 medium
pineapple	1 round centre slice
plums	2 medium
pomegranate	½ large

Starch Group

Per serving: 15 grams of carbohydrate, 2 grams of protein, and 70 calories. Whole grain and enriched breads and cereals, along with dried beans and peas, are sources of iron and thiamin. Whole grain products contain more fibre than those made from refined flours. Folacin and potassium are found in many starchy vegetables.

BREADS

bagel	½ small
bread (loaf, average size slice)	1 slice
French, granary, pumpernickel, raisin, rye, white, whole wheat	
scone, 2 inch/5 cm*	1
breadcrumbs, dry	3 T.
muffin	½
hamburger bun	½
hot dog roll	½
pancake, 6 inch/15 cm diameter*	1
pizza crust	⅛ slice from 8 inch/20 cm pizza
roll, plain	1 small
tortilla, 6 inch/15 cm diameter	1
waffle, 5 inch × ½*	1
wheat, thin sliced	2 slices

*Omit 1 FAT serving.

CEREALS
    pearl barley   1½ T.
    bran, unprocessed   4 T.
    bulgur, cooked   4 oz/100 g
    cereal, cooked   4 oz/100 g
    cereal, dry:
        All Bran   1 oz/25 g
        Bran Flakes   ¾ oz/20 g
        Corn Flakes   ¾ oz/20 g
        Grapenuts   ¾ oz/ 20 g
        Rolled Oats   ¾ oz/20 g
        Puffed Rice   ¾ oz/20 g
        Puffed Wheat   1 oz/25 g
        Raisin Bran   ¾ oz/20 g
        Rice Krispies   1 oz/25 g
        Shredded Wheat   1 biscuit
        Special K   ¾ oz/20 g
        Wheat Flakes   ¾ oz/20 g
    flour   2½ T.
    pasta, cooked   2 oz/50 g
    popcorn (popped without added fat)   1½ oz/35 g
    rice or barley, cooked 2 oz/50 g
    wheat germ, plain   1 oz/25 g

UNSWEETENED CRACKERS
    bath oliver   1¼
    butter puff, Crawfords* 1½
    cream crackers, Jacobs 2
    crispbread, average   2
    matzoth, 6×4 inch/15×10 cm ½
    melba toast   4
    Ritz crackers, Nabisco 4
    snack crackers, Nabisco 2½
    water biscuits, Carr's, large 2½
          small   5

*Omit 1 FAT serving.

BEANS

baked beans (with tomato sauce)	3½ oz/80 g
dried beans, cooked – red kidney, soy, butter;	2 oz/50 g
black-eyed, cow, split peas, lentils	2½ oz/65 g

STARCHY VEGETABLES

broad beans	4 oz/100 g
sweetcorn	3 oz/75 g
corn on the cob, 6 inch/15 cm	½
frozen mixed (rice, peas and mushrooms)	2 oz/50 g
parsnips	4 oz/100 g
peas, green	3½ oz/80 g
potato	1 small
potato, mashed, without fat or milk	2 oz/50 g
pumpkin	4½ oz/125 g

PREPARED FOODS

angel food cake	1 small slice, *or* 1½ inch/3 cm cube
crisps, potato or corn†	15
potatoes, french fried*	8
sorbet, fruit ice	2 oz/50 g

Meat Group

All these foods are excellent sources of protein and many are good sources of iron, zinc, vitamin B_{12}, and other B vitamins. Try to limit your intake of red meat, increasing instead poultry and fish. The latter contain smaller amounts of cholesterol. Remember that the following three meat groups are slightly different and that at least 2 of your 3 daily meat *portions* (breakfast, lunch and dinner) should come from the low fat, group A meats.

* Omit 1 FAT serving.
† Omit 2 FAT servings.

All canned fish should be packed in water or brine. Meats should be trimmcd of all visible fat. Have beef trimmed before mincing. Cook without added fat.

LOW FAT
Each serving contains 7 grams of protein, 3 grams of fat, and 55 calories.

Beef
chuck steak	1 oz/25 g
flank	1 oz/25 g
skirt	1 oz/25 g
tripe	1 oz/25 g

Cheese
cottage, low-fat	2 oz/50 g
curd, skim milk, 2 per cent fat	3 oz/75 g
other low-fat cheeses, less than 5 per cent butterfat	3 T.

Fish
any fish, fresh or frozen	1 oz/25 g
shellfish, fresh or frozen	1 oz/25 g
fish or shellfish, canned	3 oz/75 g
sardines, drained	3 medium

Frog legs   1 oz/25 g

Lamb
all cuts except breast	1 oz/25 g

Pork
leg	1 oz/25 g
raw continental or smoked ham, all cuts	1 oz/25 g

Poultry (without skin)
boiling fowl	1 oz/25 g

135

chicken	1 oz/25 g
pheasant	1 oz/25 g
turkey	1 oz/25 g

Rabbit   1 oz/25 g

Tofu (soybean curd)   2½ oz/65 g

Veal
all cuts except breast   1 oz/25 g

Venison   1 oz/25 g

MEDIUM FAT
Each serving contains 7 grams of protein, 5 grams of fat, and 75 calories.

Beef

corned beef (canned)	1 oz/25 g
porterhouse steak	1 oz/25 g
sirloin steak	1 oz/25 g
T-bone steak	1 oz/25 g
tongue	1 oz/25 g
wing or best rib	1 oz/25 g

Cheese

cottage, with added cream	2 oz/50 g
low-fat curd	1 oz/25 g
Neufchâtel	1 oz/25 g
processed spread	1 oz/25 g

Eggs   1

Organ meats

heart	1 oz/25 g
kidney	1 oz/25 g
liver	1 oz/25 g

sweetbreads   1 oz/25 g

Pork
  gammon or bacon joint   1 oz/25 g
  ham (cooked, canned)   1 oz/25 g
  loin (all chops, blade, chine,
      chump roast)   1 oz/25 g
  hand and spring   1 oz/25 g
  forehock   1 oz/25 g

HIGH FAT*
Each serving contains 7 grams of protein, 8 grams of fat, and
100 calories.

Beef
  Brisket   1 oz/25 g
  minced beef, commercial   1 oz/25 g

Cheese
  All hard and semi-hard cheeses, soft
  full-fat and quick-ripening cheeses,
  and blue cheeses, e.g., cheddar,
  Edam, Boursin, Brie, Camembert,
  Danish Blue and Stilton. Also
  processed cheeses.   1 oz/25 g

Cold delicatessen meats and sausages   1 oz/25 g

Hot dog   1 oz/25 g
                                           (½ average)

Lamb
  breast, rolled roast, braised or stewed 1 oz/25 g

Peanut butter   1½ T.

  * Omit 1 FAT serving for each of the following items.

Pork and bacon

back or streaky bacon rashers	1 oz/25 g
pork spareribs	1 oz/25 g
loin, chump, hock	1 oz/25 g

Poultry

duck (domestic)	1 oz/25 g
goose	1 oz/25 g

Sausage	1 chipolata or 2 cocktail sausages

Veal

breast (as lamb)	1 oz/25 g

Vegetable Group*

Per serving: 5 grams of carbohydrate, 2 grams of protein, and 25 calories.

Dark green and deep yellow vegetables are terrific sources of vitamin A. Use different vegetables each day to get vitamin C, folacin, and B_6. All vegetables contain fibre.

FREE: Eat these as you desire.

chicory	all types of lettuce
Chinese cabbage	parsley
endive	radishes

RESTRICTED

alfalfa sprouts 1 oz/25 g	brussels sprouts 4 oz/100 g
globe artichoke 1 medium	cabbage 4 oz/100 g
asparagus 4-6 medium spears	carrots 1 medium
aubergine 6 oz/175 g	cauliflower florets 6 oz/175 g
bean sprouts, mung 2 oz/50 g	celery 3 small stalks
beans, green 1½ oz/35 g	courgettes 5 oz/150 g
beetroot 2 medium	cucumber 6 oz/175 g
broccoli 3 spears	greens:

*Starchy vegetables are included in the Starch Group.

beetroot tops 3 oz/75 g
Swiss chard 3 oz/75 g
kale 3 oz/75 g
spinach 3 oz/75 g
turnip tops 3 oz/75 g
leeks 2 oz/50 g
marrow 5 oz/150 g
mushrooms 3 oz/75 g
okra 8-9 pods
onions 3½ oz/85 g

pepper, green or red
  1 medium
rhubarb 12 oz/340 g
sauerkraut 4 oz/100 g
swedes 3½ oz/85 g
tomato juice 4 fl oz/120 ml
tomatoes 5 oz/150 g
turnips 4 oz/100 g
vegetable juice cocktail
  4 fl oz/120 ml

Fat Group
Per serving: 5 grams of fat and 45 calories. Since these are concentrated sources of calories, they must be measured especially carefully. Try to use fats of vegetable rather than animal origin, because they are lower in saturated fat and higher in unsaturated fat. (See page 199 for an explanation.)

avocado	¾ oz/30 g
bacon	1 rasher
bacon fat	1 tsp.
butter	1½ tsp.
low-calorie spread	3 tsp.
chocolate, cooking	2 tsp. *or* ⅓ oz/8 g
coconut, desiccated	2 T.
cocoa, dry powder	3 T.
cream:	
pouring or coffee	3 T.
double	1 T.
double, whipped	2 T.
single	2 T.
soured	2 T.
full fat cheese	1 T.
lard	1 tsp.
margarine	1½ tsp.
mayonnaise	1 tsp.

mayonnaise, low calorie	2 tsp.
nuts:	
almonds	10 whole
macadamia	3
peanuts	20 whole
pecans, large	2
pistachios	20
other	6
oil	1 tsp.
olives, green or black	5 small

Salad dressing	
blue cheese, any type	2 tsp.
French	1 T.
mayonnaise-type	1 T.
Russian	2 tsp.
Thousand Island	2 tsp.
tartare sauce	1 T.

Miscellaneous

Per serving: 0 or negligible calories. Eat as desired (except where noted).

artificial sweetener
stock cubes (clear fat-free* *or* low-sodium)
soda water* (low-sodium *or* fat-free brands)
coffee†
gelatine, sugar-free or unflavoured
chewing gum, sugar-free
herbs
horseradish
lemon
lime
mineral water

---

* All high in salt. Keep it to one pickle and 2 glasses of any of these drinks daily, unless your doctor advises less.

† High in caffeine (see page 204), so you may want to limit your intake.

mustard (use ketchup sparingly)
pickles: dill or sour*
soft drinks, sugar-free*
spices
tea†
vinegar†

Alcohol

Count alcohol as a FAT. The calories in alcohol can be calculated: $0.8 \times \text{proof} \times \text{ounces} = \text{calories}$. Each 45 calories should be counted as 1 FAT serving. Dry wines and light beers are good choices. Liqueurs and sweet mixed drinks contain considerable quantities of sugar and should be avoided.

---

* All high in salt. Keep it to one pickle and 2 glasses of any of these drinks daily, unless your doctor advises less.

† High in caffeine (see page 204), so you may want to limit your intake.

12. The Walkout –
Easier Than a Workout

You're probably a little sceptical about this walking business. You've been on a diet before, and I'm sure mine makes sense to you. But *walking*? I bet that secretly you don't believe it will work.

But this is a fact: in a university study, overweight women who made no change in their eating habits but walked at least thirty minutes a day lost an average of twenty-two pounds per year.

Next you're going to be telling me you really need spot-reducing. And I'll tell you there is no such thing. In a study at the University of Massachusetts, twenty-one people involved in a rigorous programme of sit-ups were found to have lost a small amount of fat from their middles – but also from their backs and backsides. Exercise doesn't help you lose weight from a specific spot.

Women put on weight in a predetermined fashion: first on the back of the thigh, then the inside, and next, in order, hips, midriff, and upper body (such as arms). Fat will decrease in reverse order from the way it was put on – no matter what specific exercise you do. By working on a specific muscle as you do in a sit-up, you just develop that muscle and make it larger, while the fat stays on top of it. Only aerobic exercise, which draws fat equally from every part of the body, will help change your shape.

Next you're going to be telling me you already walk a lot. A plump friend of mine from Los Angeles used to tell me that she was a great walker. She came along with me one day – I'd been walking for about four months at the time – and I kept my usual pace, or perhaps even a bit slower. After the walk, we went different ways, and then I called her later in the afternoon to confirm our dinner plans. She had to cancel: she'd taken to her bed with exhaustion.

Let me tell you something. If you really *are* walking a lot, then you don't have a fat problem. If you do, then you only *think* you're walking a lot.

Why walking and not weightlifting. There are two kinds of exercises. One kind, such as weightlifting, sprinting, golf, even callisthenics, is stop-and-start exercising. The other is continuous exercise – such as jogging, dancing and walking. Exercise in this category is considered 'aerobic'.

'Aerobic' exercise uses oxygen. During the course of aerobic exercise, your heart beats faster, your lungs expand, and your blood vessels open up in order to carry blood loaded with oxygen to the cells. The more oxygen you use, the more fat gets burned. The most popular aerobic exercises are swimming, bicycling, skipping rope, dancing, jogging, and walking.

What to tell your friends when they recommend jogging. Lots of folks aren't that crazy about the alternatives to walking. I'm not. Take swimming: you have to change out of your clothes into your suit, then back again. It takes up a lot of time. Then you get your hair wet, and either you get one of those short haircuts or you arrive back at your office with a fresh-out-of-the-sauna look. I don't know about you, but I don't think I'm blonde or Nordic enough for that. A skipping rope doesn't interest me. I've tried bicycling, but that's not much fun in the winter. Besides, once you're on your bike, you're committed to it. Suppose you feel like walking back? I've tried a stationary bicycle, but I feel the way I do when I take gas at the dentist's office: time is standing still. Dancing is nice, but I remember being asked to sign a medical release when I signed up for class. I think that if you're not in shape, it's just too much. Besides, I know you aren't too anxious to get into a leotard when you feel more like a wreckette than a Rockette.

And then there's jogging. Now, I've tried it, as I

mentioned, and I didn't like it. For one thing, I find it aesthetically unappealing to see big women jogging. Besides, I don't think it's natural for human beings. Animals do it, but animals move on all fours.

In fact, I see that scientists have a lot of animals out jogging these days. A bunch of jogging monkeys were used in research to determine if people who exercised would have arteries that were less clogged than those who didn't. There was even a group of 'Yucatan mini swine' – that's pigs, to you and me – who were running a hundred miles a week around a San Diego laboratory to prove that exercise could be beneficial even if your arteries were clogged. (It seems to be; but walking is exercise, too.) I prefer to leave the jogging to animals; they do very well at it.

Jogging can also lead to problems – skeletal injuries, foot problems, organ displacement, stress fractures, sprains and breaks. Even eye problems, like detached retinas, and ear problems connected with balance are linked to jogging. Moreover, as you get older, the situation gets worse. Your ligaments and tendons lose their flexibility, making it easier to break limbs, dislocate joints and tear muscles. You might end up a perfect cardiovascular specimen using a cane.

And here's, so to speak, a kick in the teeth: it seems that if you jog without a bra, your breasts can slap against you with as much as seventy pounds of pressure.

It also turns out that walking five miles may take longer than jogging five miles but they both burn off the same number of calories.

Walking definitely works to make you lean and fit. In many ways it seems to be the best exercise you can do. Here are some of the reasons:

1. Walking is easy. I have actually read books that include instructions on how to walk, but almost everyone I've met past the age of about fourteen months seems to have it down pat.

2. Walking is cheap, particularly since you're supposed to be walking too fast to window-shop.
3. You can't hurt yourself. Well, I suppose you could, but why aren't you looking where you're going?
4. You can camouflage yourself. I now believe that thin people probably thought, at least she's trying to do something about herself, but I used to think they considered me a comical sight when I was out exercising. Still, no out-of-shape person likes to draw attention – but you can walk in the middle of crowds.
5. It's efficient. You can transport yourself and exercise yourself at the same time. Look at the fuel you're saving. I was toying with the idea of just throwing away my car keys.
6. You don't have to change clothes to walk, and you won't need a shower and another change to look presentable whenever you get where you're going.

The Walkout – How to Do It

Frequency
At least five times a week. A 1980 study showed that exercise four and five times a week is three times as effective as exercise three times a week. Exercise once or twice a week is almost useless. *Also, don't skip two days in a row.*

Time of Day
Before a meal or up to one hour after. There is some indication that fat storage pathways are more efficient at night, so it *may* be helpful to exercise then. If you've done your aerobic exercise before eating, you may want to take a little extra, moderate walk directly after eating to take advantage of dietary thermogenesis. (Even if you do your aerobic exercise as much as an hour after a meal, you will still take advantage of dietary thermogenesis.)

Help Yourself: the Programme

Amount

Start at twenty minutes and work up to sixty. Take it slow for the first couple of weeks: start with twenty minutes per day, then go up to thirty. You're out of shape and I can't promise you this will be fun. It won't be aerobic either, since that requires at least thirty minutes of continuous exercise plus warm-up time. Walking during the first two weeks is just meant to get you out of the door.

Remember: walking is not a punishment. It becomes a routine, like brushing your teeth, but, it also becomes a pleasure. You will start looking forward to your walk.

Do not over-exert in the first few days. You may decide you can do better than you're supposed to. Don't get so carried away that you spend the next couple of days lying in bed with warm towels to recuperate. You've destroyed the whole purpose of the walking, which is that it must be done regularly.

Dr Joel told me to set aside an hour a day for walking. The hour could *include* ten minutes of warm-up and ten of cool down, he said, but I'd be better off doing the warm-up in addition to an hour of brisk walking. At the end of this section, you'll find some warm-up exercises. As for cooling down, you do that simply by slowing down your pace. When you're walking at top speed, you're using your heart to pump extra blood into your arms and legs. If you stop too abruptly, you may get some cramping.

Not until you've walked quickly, for at least thirty minutes, does fat burning take place. As you know, the body first burns carbohdyrates for energy, and only after it uses them up does it go to the fat stores.

Speed

Until you're moving at 70 per cent of maximum heart rate. You saw the word per cent and figured you weren't going to like this part, right? Numbers are not something I'm fond of, either. They bring up unpleasant associations: how many pounds on the scale, how many inches around my thigh, how many calories in this portion. But please bear with me; I have to talk about numbers here.

Dr Joel pointed out to me that when he said to walk, he meant *move*. You're not supposed to be window-shopping; you're supposed to be pretending that Norman Bates from *Psycho* is after you. Walk with a purpose: you do have one, of course.

The best way to gauge yourself is to take your own pulse.

For the wrist pulse: press the first two fingers of your right hand (if you're right-handed) across the opposite forearm, about an inch above the wrist. Press hard enough to feel the thumping of the blood but not so hard that you block it off. Time yourself using a clock with a second hand. Count the first beat as zero.

For the neck pulse: this might be easier for you. Place the first three fingers of your hand just below the angle of the jaw. Stretch your neck out, and move your fingers slowly down your neck until you feel the beat. *Do not press* – you're supposed to *feel* the beat, not halt it. Press too hard and you'll cut off the blood supply.

Do you remember hearing that 72 was the perfect pulse rate? Most Americans' pulses are in the eighties and nineties, but someone in good condition can have a pulse rate of 65 or lower.

How hard you're exercising is determined by how fast your pulse is moving. The rate you strive for is calculated after you've figured out your maximum pulse rate.

To find your maximum pulse rate, subtract your age from the number 220. If you're 40, your maximum rate is 180 $(220-40 = 180)$. Of course, you don't exercise to the maximum. Right now I'm sure you couldn't. And if you could, you would pass out fairly soon. Athletes in excellent shape push themselves to about 85 per cent and you should strive for about 70 per cent.

If your maximum pulse rate is 180, multiply that by 70 per cent and you'll see that your exercise rate should be 126 $(180 \times 70 = 126)$.

EXERCISE HEART RATES

Age	Maximum Rate	10-second count (70 per cent of maximum)	Age	Maximum Rate	10-second count (70 per cent of maximum)
18	202	24	45	175	20
19	201	23	46	174	20
20	200	23	47	173	20
21	199	23	48	172	20
22	198	23	49	171	20
23	197	23	50	170	20
24	196	23	51	169	20
25	195	23	52	168	20
26	194	23	53	167	19
27	193	23	54	166	19
28	192	22	55	165	19
29	191	22	56	164	19
30	190	22	57	163	19
31	189	22	58	162	19
32	188	22	59	161	19
33	187	22	60	160	19
34	186	22	61	159	19
35	185	22	62	158	18
36	184	21	63	157	18
37	183	21	64	156	18
38	182	21	65	155	18
39	181	21	66	154	18
40	180	21	67	153	18
41	179	21	68	152	18
42	178	21	69	151	18
43	177	20	70	150	18
44	176	20			

I suggest you find out what your ten-second rate should be (in this case it's 21, since 21×6 = 126). This is because while you're out walking and checking your pulse, it's more efficient to stop for only ten seconds rather than a minute. With the above chart, I've spared you the trouble of figuring this out for yourself.

After the first five to ten minutes of exercising, you should get up to 50 per cent of maximum rate. The worse shape you're in, the faster it will get there.

I know you'll be tempted to stop much too often to check your pulse, so here's a rule-of-thumb test to see if you've reached your 70 per cent of maximum level. If you can carry on a conversation or – just barely – manage to sing out loud, you're probably going along at the right speed.

Just remember: the more you walk, and the faster you walk, the quicker that weight will come off and the faster you'll shape up.

Distance
3½ or 4 miles per hour is what you're striving for.

The major reason you're walking is to rebuild the lean muscle mass in your body and increase thermogenesis, but remember you're also walking to burn up calories. The way to gauge that is to find out how much ground you've covered.

The figure of calories burned is only an estimate because the number is influenced by several factors including weight, age, sex, general fitness, and the genetic variations between individuals.

Scientists figure out how many calories you burn by measuring how much oxygen you use. If you use one litre of oxygen, you burn 4.82 calories a minute. So if a seven-stone person uses a third of a litre of oxygen in a minute of dishwashing, she uses up a third of 4.8, or about 1.6 calories per minute.

The more frequently and more deeply you breathe during exercise, the more oxygen you use; and the more oxygen you use, the more calories you burn.

Here's a guide to measure how many calories you're burning an hour. Multiply your weight (in pounds) times the figure below:

If you're walking 2 miles per hour, multiply your weight by 1.30

2¼	1.56
3	1.80
3¼	2.05
4	2.35
4¼	3.10
5	3.85

In other words, if you weigh 200 lb and you're going 2 miles per hour, you're burning 260 calories (1.30×200).

How fast you go is partly determined by the length of your legs, too: a short-legged person might find a pace of 20 minutes per mile or 3 miles per hour moderate and 15 minutes per mile or 4 miles per hour fast, while a taller person might manage a 17-minute mile moving moderately and an 11–12-minute mile moving quickly.

That's it. That's all you have to know. Just get out there and start walking.

Warm-up Exercises

I'm suggesting a few, but there are quite a number of variations that would be acceptable. Perhaps you even have an old exercise book lying around the house that you always meant to do something about. Use it. Or follow these:

Loosening Up

1. Stand tall, with your feet about 12 inches/30 cm apart. Breathe deeply in and out. Ten times in all.
2. Stand tall. Stick arms straight out. Make ten pumpkin-size circles forward, then ten in reverse. Repeat.
3. Stand tall. Close eyes, relax jaw, drop your head forward. Rotate your head ten times clockwise, then ten times counterclockwise.
4. Stand tall. Rotate shoulders forward ten times, then backwards ten times.

Stretching

1. Toes. Sit on floor with legs in front of you straight out. Keep heels on the floor. Point your toes all the way forward and hold for a count of ten, then point your toes towards your body, hold for a count of ten. Fifteen times for each foot.

2. Ankles. Remain sitting, with legs straight out. Lift your foot and rotate your ankle, making large circles ten times in one direction, then ten in reverse direction. Repeat with other foot.

3. Feet. Sit on floor cross-legged, left foot on top of right thigh. Grab the foot with both hands, the sole in the left hand, the top with the right hand. Don't move your leg or your knee; just bend the ankle. Then twist your foot so that the sole points upward and you feel a pull. Hold for a count of ten. Repeat with other foot.

4. Calves. Stand at arm's length from a wall. Stretch one leg out behind you, keeping the knee straight. Slightly bend the knee of the forward leg. Keeping both heels on the floor, lean in against the wall until you feel a pull. Hold for a count of fifteen. Repeat with other leg. Do this eight times with each leg.

5. Front of thigh. Stand. Hold your right heel in your right hand and pull gently. If you can, pull the foot up to touch your hip. Hold for a count of ten. Repeat with other leg. Five times for each leg.

6. Back of thigh. Put your right foot on a table about three feet high. Now bend over and reach for your left toes with both hands. Keep legs and back straight. Feel the pull in the back of your thighs and lower back. Hold for a count of ten. Repeat with other leg. Ten times for each leg.

7. Whole body. Put your feet two feet apart and bend forward, stretching from lower back. Grab your right ankle with both hands and bring your face down to your knee. Hold for a count of ten. Repeat with other leg. Five times for each leg.

Weather or Not

Rain

You wake up, take a look out the window, and see it's raining. You think, great! At least I don't have to do that walking stuff today. You're wrong. Today is a day like any other. Get out there. Put on your raincoat and go through that front door. Now I'm not suggesting you go out into a tornado, but a little rain never hurt anyone. If you get yourself a good anorak and some comfortable boots, the rain won't even bother you. Still, if you can't stand the sound of mud oozing underfoot, let me remind you that there are some places you can walk indoors.

- Shopping malls. Almost every city has one. Just don't stop where they're selling food. You're not supposed to stop while you're walking anyway. You might plan to have your fourth meal and a cup of black coffee when the hour's over.
- Indoor tracks. You'd be surprised at how many clubs and schools have tracks available for public use. Let your fingers do the walking to locate a place where your legs can do the walking.
- Airports. I don't mean the runway. I mean inside. Airports in major cities are huge. Going from one end to the other is a great way to kill time and keep you out of the cocktail lounge.
- Museums. Walk through at a brisk pace. Don't feel strange. Just pretend you're looking for someone. This may prove to be a problem if it rains for several days on end: the security guards become suspicious. On the other hand, you might get a reputation as a real art lover. Make sure that during your cool down, when you're going a little more slowly, you actually do look at what's on the walls or in the cases. Someone might ask you about the current show.

One place I wouldn't suggest you do your walking: a supermarket.

You might want some suggestions for equipment:

- Waterproof. Keep a fold-up jacket with you at all times. Get something with a hood. I don't know about you, but I never feel as if I can really *move* with an umbrella.
- Boots. Make sure they're waterproof. Wet feet cause blisters, aside from feeling awful.

Keep thinking how great the rain is for your skin. English beauties, famous for their clear complexions, are said to get them from walking through the mists on the moors.

Cold

Don't tell me you can't walk in the cold. I do, and I live in Minneapolis, where even the ground hogs don't come out in February. Get into your coat and your mittens and remind yourself how cute you look when your face is flushed from the cold.

- Bonus: moderately overweight people who do aerobic exercise in cold weather burn extra fat.
- Walk into the wind (it's colder) at the beginning of your walk, and away from it as you return.
- Skin freezes at 25° F/−3° C and below. You might want to consider wearing a ski mask if it's really frigid out.
- Wear a hat. You lose a great deal of your body heat through your head.
- Your battery-operated cassette player may go on the fritz in the cold, since the low temperature slows down the chemical action used to make electricity. Keep it under heavy clothes and close to your body. Once you're indoors, the power will return to normal.

153

Hot Weather

- A lightweight hat soaked in water and squeezed dry might help keep you cool.
- Drink extra water. This not only prevents heat exhaustion but if you become dehydrated, your body confuses thirst and hunger and you become ravenous.
- If you have muscle cramps in your legs, that may indicate that you need more potassium – which is lost, together with sodium, when you sweat. Drink 8 fl oz of skim milk; eat a fruit that's high in potassium, such as melons, bananas, oranges or apricots, or choose a potato at dinner.

Shoes

I have bought many pairs of walking shoes, but not until 1982 did I actually wear out a pair. I used to think of them as cruel shoes, but now I don't go anywhere without them. If I go to a formal do I have them in a bag in my car. A few words about shoes:

- Use running shoes for walking. Nylon uppers are good for hot weather because they allow circulation; and leather uppers are good in rainy and snowy weather. They keep out wetness, which causes blisters.
- Remove scuffs on white leather uppers with typewriter correction fluid.
- When new ones are stiff, bend them at the ball of the foot, then tape them in that position and leave that way overnight.
- If nylon uppers on your shoes get wet, stuff them with newspapers and let dry (away from heat and direct sunlight at room temperature).

. . . And Socks

- Wear two pairs of thin socks rather than one pair of thick ones to keep in the heat and reduce the chance of getting a blister. (If you do get one, cut a piece of foam into a square, cut a hole in the foam, and tape it over the blister.)

- Buy a pair of silk socks to put under your other ones. They're terrific for keeping the heat in.

Equipment
- One other piece of equipment you might enjoy: a pedometer.
- Or you could treat yourself to a Japanese-made Jogger Mate Pulse Meter. About the size of a business card, it's a little boxlike gizmo with a moving needle which registers your pulse.
- Major splurge: a treadmill. I have one and it's the greatest. (Now I know somebody is going to ask how come I hate stationary bicycles and love my treadmill. On both of them, you're going nowhere; but on a stationary bicycle you're going there faster. What's the rush?)

How to Get Yourself Going: Buy a Portable Cassette Player You Can Wear on Your Waist
There's nothing like music with a beat to get you going. I started off with 'Sixteen Tons' and now I'm ready to move to 'The Flight of the Bumblebee'. You can listen to your favourite music, of course, but there are other special things you can do with your player and headphones:

- Tape the soap operas while you're doing something else around the house, then catch up with them while you're out walking the next day. You may have to use your imagination during some of the quiet spots, but that might be a plus.
- Buy a tape that helps you learn a foreign language.
- Instead of writing a letter to someone, tape your message while you walk, and ask for a taped letter in reply.
- Tape a speech you have to give and play it back so you can memorize it.
- While your head is clear, record a list of all the things you have to accomplish – short-term or long-term.

155

- Learn the lyrics to songs you always wanted to be able to sing along with.
- Listen to a tape recording of a play instead of music for a change. You can probably borrow one from your library.

I'd Rather Walk Alone

You're going to read here and there about how you should organize groups of friends, neighbours and colleagues to walk with you. I think this is a big bunch of baloney. The first rainy day that comes along, they'll all cop out on you. My friends did. They didn't have my fat problem and so they didn't have the motivation that I did – and you will.

I know sometimes you'll find it difficult to keep on walking, but remember that you have to work very hard to be normal again. One of my good friends, a woman who always has had a terrific body, promised to come along with me one day and sure enough, the weather was rotten and she decided to stay home. So there I was with my parka on, and my hat and my ear muffs and my gloves, pushing along and feeling really sorry for myself. Why me? I was thinking. Why do I have to work this hard? Of course, I was sure I was the only one suffering the way I was. Then I got out to the lake and there were dozens of people out there doing the same thing I was, either to get in shape or stay in shape. (If you have a vengeful streak, maybe it will make you feel better to think that someday it'll catch up with them. The friends sitting home will be huffing and puffing at some future date to work off those extra pounds they're putting on now.)

Enjoy being out there and being by yourself. At least you don't have to listen to Joe Blow's office politics or the marital saga of Sally Smith.

Another bonus: the sound of silence. If you've spent most of your life trying to tune out the din of an office or assorted kids, pets and other loved ones, you might find you're crazy about being alone with yourself. Walking gives you some time alone that you'd probably otherwise find impossible to get. If you get too lonely, just turn on your portable cassette player and let your favourite D.J. entertain you.

Walking Not Only Makes You Fit and Lean, but Also

- Improves your circulation. Your hands and feet won't get as cold as they used to.
- Reduces your chances of getting osteoporosis, a bone disease not uncommon in older women, since increased strength, fitness and activity help prevent weak bones.
- Lessens the chance of hardening of the arteries by increasing HDL cholesterol, a blood protein that transports the other kind of cholesterol out of the artery walls. That makes you less susceptible to a stroke or heart attack in later middle age and old age.
- Stimulates you to secrete sleep-inducing endorphins. You'll have the soundest sleep you've ever had. Now I find I don't sleep unless I've walked. So I've got two motivators: staying fit and sleeping. Otherwise I might be up all night eating.
- Helps prevent the kind of diabetes that's common in middle age.
- Improves your posture, which results in fewer back pains, aching legs, and varicose veins and also builds abdominal muscles.
- Lets you walk your problems away. You may not get rid of them, but you'll sure get the tension out of your system.

13. Mary Ellen's Forty-four Best Diet Tips

1. Make a Doctor's Appointment and Keep It

You've read this warning in every diet book you've ever read.

> **WARNING**
> Do not embark on this or any other
> diet programme without first
> consulting your physician.

But you didn't, did you? You knew if you marched in there with that cockamamie diet you last went on your doctor would have laughed you right out of the office. Well, I'm telling you to see your doctor, and I mean it. I'm not saying it as a disclaimer so that if something goes wrong, I won't get in hot water. I'm saying it so something goes right. If you're in the same shape as I was before I went to Dr Joel, you're probably long overdue for a check-up anyway. Just make sure the doctor is someone you can trust. And who knows? Maybe you'll be one of the lucky ones and it will turn out your weight problem is a thyroid condition after all.

2. Quit Procrastinating

I know all the excuses. I've used them myself. I once put off starting my next diet until the coming of Halley's Comet. As you may recall, Halley's Comet comes around once in every seventy-six years and it had been seen the day before I made my vow. There is no rule that you have to wait until Monday to start a diet, or until after the holidays: it won't be a less joyful Christmas if you're not stuffing yourself along with the goose. If you're the way I was, when you're not dieting, you're gaining. The longer you put the diet off, the fatter you're going to be when you finally start it. So pick up the phone and make a doctor's appointment *now*, and before you get there finish this book and start planning your walking schedule. (You can buy your walking shoes and diet groceries on the way home from the doctor's office.)

3. Forget Being a Big Beautiful Doll Unless You Are One

You've seen the models in the large-size clothing catalogues. They weigh fourteen stone and more, their bodies are firm as the Rock of Gibraltar, and they look great. But I don't think the average shopper in the places that cater for larger women is cover girl material. If I had looked like a Big Beautiful Doll, I'd have been proud; but the only modelling agency that would have hired me at fifteen stone was an outfit called Funny Face. If you're big and beautiful, all you have to do is start looking for larger men to look good next to. But I don't think there are too many Big Beautiful Guys out there either.

4. Eat Meals on Regular-Size Plates

I don't believe in the school of thought that says you should put your food on doll plates so you think there's more of it. You'd better learn what 6 oz/175 g chicken looks like so you can gauge what you're eating anywhere. And that advice about always leaving something on your plate leaves me cold, too. If you're not supposed to be eating it, what's it doing on your plate anyway?

5. Write Down Whatever You Eat

And I mean *everything*. The dab of butter here, the bite of apple there. All that stuff that adds up to a few billion calories if you don't keep track. On page 250, there's a sample diary page. Make yourself a few photocopies and tuck them in your bag along with a pencil. Be as faithful in keeping a record as you were with your first diary.

6. If You're Having a Craving, Wait Twenty Minutes Before You Give In

There it is: that piece of cake left over from your son's birthday party. You want it, don't you? Stop. First drink a glass of water, then find something else to do for twenty minutes. Walk. Read a book. Call an old boyfriend. Nine out of ten times, the urge will have passed. Whatever was luring you with its siren call won't seem too appealing after you've delayed the gratification.

. . . And if you eat it after all, then go out and walk for fifteen minutes.

So you ate it. I hope it tasted good. Now forget it, stop guilt-tripping, and leave the house. Take a fifteen-minute bonus walk. You just turned a negative situation into a positive one. As you walk, remind yourself, 'I'll do better next time.'

7. To Err Is Human, to Binge Divine

Let's face it. You're going to cheat once in a while. I did, and that's normal. I must tell you it got easier to stay on the programme once I started getting results; also, after a while I lost my desire for some of the junk that had tempted me in the past. But there were occasions when I went out to dinner or to a party and went a little overboard. In some cases, I jumped ship entirely. The next morning, I'd get up, and instead of starting the day with a block of Dairy Mint Choc Chip ice cream, I'd eat my normal breakfast, do my walking, and just get back on the programme. (I didn't cut back because I slipped, either.) Most diets fail because someone says, 'I ate too much last night; I've ruined everything anyway.'

8. Eat Four Times a Day

I thought I was doing myself a favour when I skipped breakfast. If I wasn't hungry, why should I eat? I always viewed breakfast as extra, useless calories. I often skipped lunch, too. By dinnertime, I wanted something really substantial, like a tree. I started at six o'clock and kept on going, with occasional breaks, until midnight. Now I know it's important to eat regularly. You get less hungry, so you don't gorge. Besides, when you eat, you start dietary thermogenesis, the process in which your body burns extra calories just in the act of processing foods. When you don't eat, you miss out on this process and reduce your metabolism rate, too. It may be called *fasting*, but it actually slows you down.

9. Eating Between Meals

Let's be honest. There isn't a doggy-bag in the world big enough to carry around all the food you really want. When you're eating a carrot stick, you don't want a carrot stick. You want a nice big hunk of chocolate cake.

Why should I tell you to carry an apple around if you get hungry between meals? Do I think you're going to say, 'What a great idea! I'll have an apple instead of a candy bar'? If you were the kind of person who chooses apples between meals, you wouldn't be overweight in the first place.

All you're doing with the carrot and the celery and the apples is substituting one kind of eating for another. And what you should be doing is training yourself to eat only at meals. If you're following the programme properly, you shouldn't be hungry between meals anyway.

10. Don't Eat to Pep Yourself Up

Most of us think if we eat a little something, we'll feel better. If we're feeling blah, food will give us instant energy. Think about it. 'Energetic' is not a word often applied to people who are eating all the time. Eating is not a cure-all.

If you're feeling dizzy and tired, get out of the kitchen and into bed so you don't fall over the stove or into the refrigerator and hurt yourself. I'm joking, but the point is, if you're eating properly, you won't get dizzy and tired in the first place. Next time you're about to make a little excursion into the fridge, stop for a moment and ask if you're experiencing true hunger.

Do you just want junk food? Have you had a real meal within the past two hours? Has something upset you or made you happy? What you're feeling isn't hunger.

Or have you skipped a meal? Has it been four hours since you've eaten? Would you be satisfied with a nutritious meal instead of junk food? Is your stomach growling? Do you feel really empty? Any of these symptoms means you're feeling true hunger, and it's time for a meal.

11. Put Your Fork Down Between Bites

Put your spoon and knife down, too. Straws aren't allowed either. Have a little conversation during the meal. Don't dive into your food. Watch thin people eat. They sometimes hold something on their fork and forget about it while they talk. Bet you never did that.

Did you know that speed eaters can consume three courses in twenty gulps? Twenty dips and it's all over. They're like high-powered vacuum cleaners. You have to learn to be a carpet sweeper.

Here's how you do it. For lunch, plan to eat for thirty minutes. For dinner, plan on thirty to forty-five. Put the fork down with each bite. Chew each mouthful eight to ten times. Swallow and count four seconds before you put the fork back in your food. Do this for two days.

This is very difficult to do. I want you to know that. These meals will not go down in history as among the best you have ever eaten. In fact, the food may seem repulsive to you. That's not the point. What this is intended to do – and it will – is slow you down. It works. After a couple of days, you'll slow down automatically. You won't be counting the minutes every time you have a meal.

12. Eat at the Table

Food has always been my friend. In fact, I rarely went anywhere without it. It's even been with me in the bathroom:

olive oil on my scalp, egg yolks and mayonnaise on my face, and potato chips on my lips. The oil was to restore the natural lustre of my hair, and I used the egg yolks and mayo for a facial mask. The potato chips weren't part of the beauty treatment. They were just keeping me company.

My friend Gail's family gathers around the portable dishwasher, which serves as a snack bar, to nibble between meals. Their theory is that if you eat standing up, it doesn't count. It does, of course. Remember: elephants eat standing up.

You bought your kitchen or dining-room table to have your meals there – not just to cut out patterns on or do your kids' homework at. Try using it for its original purpose again. If you know you have to be sitting down to have a meal, you're not going to sneak in calories on the run.

13. Don't Do Anything Else While You Eat
There was a guy who couldn't walk and chew gum at the same time. He got to be President of the United States. Take a leaf from his book, and when you're chewing, don't do anything else. Eating is a legitimate activity. It deserves its own slot in your schedule. Enjoy your food. Don't grab it on the run. Don't shovel it down while you're reading the latest glossy magazine. Don't fork it in while you're watching TV; during those thrillers, it can really go down fast. When you concentrate on something else, you forget you're eating; and when you forget you're eating, you eat too much.

14. Take Pictures of Yourself Throughout the Diet
I know you don't want to look, but think of this: everyone else has to. Really. You're the only one who doesn't know how you look. You shouldn't be an ostrich with your head in the sand. Take the photos before you start your diet, and keep the picture in your head (or in your wallet) always. There is a bright side. After the first time, the pictures can only get better, and they'll help give you positive reinforcement to stay on the programme.

15. Look in Mirrors
I'm not talking about the mirror in your compact. I'm talking about a full-length mirror.

My near-sighted friend Melvyn started running when he was in his mid-forties. He was heading back to his apartment the first week at about 7.30 a.m. when he saw a peculiar figure coming towards him. He was a little nervous, but didn't think the guy would hurt him. He looked pretty bad – his face was twisted, his hair was going in every direction, and he was dressed in old clothes. 'He's probably a drug addict,' Melvyn figured. When he was about three feet away, he realized he was looking in a mirror.

I scared myself, too. Shortly before I started the diet, I went to a party and had a couple of cocktails. That gave me the courage to come home and take off my clothes and stand in front of the mirror naked. Until that moment, I thought the most terrifying thing I'd ever seen was the shark scene in *Jaws*. I can joke about it now, but it was one of the things that convinced me to go on the diet. Now I like what I see; it's one of the things that helps keep me on the programme.

16. Take Your Measurements
My overweight friend Judy was bragging about her little girl. 'She has ribs,' Judy said, 'which haven't been seen in my family for generations.' Ribs weren't the only part of my body that had gone into obscurity. I barely remembered something called 'hollows' of the neck. Even in my mind's eye, I couldn't picture what my knees looked like in the aerial view.

You'll see the difference in your clothes, but if you're like me, you need as much reinforcement as possible. So before you begin, take a deep breath and take your measurements. Actually, you'd better let that deep breath out before you look at the tape measure.

So what if your thigh measures one and a half times

Scarlett O'Hara's waist? Remember, this is the worst it's going to be. From now on, things will only get better.

Repeat the measurement as you go from step to step, or if you stay on one step for a while, measure every two weeks. You'll be surprised.

17. Weigh Only Once a Week

The most exercise I used to get was dragging the scale around the room trying to find a spot where I'd weigh the least. Who was I trying to kid? The only thing lower than fooling yourself about how much you weigh is cheating at solitaire.

Addicted dieters tend to go off the deep end if a day passes with no weight loss. 'What the hell,' they say to themselves, 'nothing much is happening so I might as well eat this side of beef.'

If you've made the commitment to the diet, you're in it for the long haul. You know your weight varies from day to day, so weigh yourself only once a week, same day, same time. And without any clothes, please; no trying to persuade yourself that your sandals weigh six pounds. If you're sticking to the programme, you'll see a loss.

18. Weigh and Measure Your Food

If you're so crazy to get at the scales, buy one to keep in the kitchen and weigh your food on it. A diet scale or even a small postal scale will do. Also, measure your food: a heaped tablespoon contains almost twice as much – and twice as many calories – as a level one.

Weighing food is the best way to learn to judge portions by sight so you can keep track of what you're eating even when you're eating out. Here's one trick that might help: a 4 oz/100 g piece of meat is about the same size as a pack of playing cards. And to gauge ¼ pint/150 ml, make a fist: this measure is about the distance from the top of your middle finger to the bottom of your little finger.

But as a rule, don't guess – weigh. If you were so good at guessing weight by looking, how could you have convinced yourself you'd only gained a couple of pounds since the last time you were on a scale . . .

19. Don't Put Yourself Down

None of those posters with pigs pasted on the refrigerator, please. None of the gadgets that say, 'You fat slob' when you open the refrigerator door. I had one of those, and I got so depressed that I went out and bought a second refrigerator. A moving man I knew once said, 'The body is just the wardrobe for the mind.' Underneath all the excess baggage is *you* – the same person who'll be there once it's gone. Start respecting yourself now, to get in practice. Imagine how good you'll feel when you've Helped Yourself.

20. Don't Be Self-Conscious

So you're fat. That's not a crime against humanity. And you're probably a nicer person because of it. Seriously: didn't most of the nicest people you know start out as goofy-looking kids? As soon as it occurs to you that your looks aren't your strong suit, if you have any brains at all you usually start developing some other drawing card. While the lookers were out on dates, the rest of us were home practising humility – or the flute.

21. Don't Obsess

Two friends of mine with some time on their hands decided to actually make the recipe for Mock Apple Pie that's on the Ritz Cracker box. You use no apples – just thirty-six Ritz Crackers. At a critical moment in the preparation, one of them discovered they were one cracker short. 'It won't work,' my other friend said. 'With thirty-five you make a Mock *Strawberry* Pie.' People on diets often think like that. If they eat three ounces instead of four, or four instead of three, the magic formula won't work.

That's not true, of course. Ideally, you follow a programme exactly. Don't keep throwing in an extra ounce here and there – it only takes sixteen to make a pound. But if you can't persuade a restaurant to serve you exactly four ounces of chicken, or you've misplaced your spoon measure and you have to guess at a half tablespoon of low-calorie mayonnaise, the world won't come to an end, and neither will your diet.

22. Shop After You've Eaten
Or you'll go through that supermarket like Pac-Man. Supermarkets are in business to make money, and they're very good at it. They know how to get your mouth watering no matter how full you are. In the old days, I used to go out and buy some sweet rolls, bring them home, sprinkle cinnamon in a little tin pan, and burn it on the stove. Once you got a whiff, you thought I'd been baking all day. That's what they do in the supermarkets. I call it Faking Baking. Don't let them fool you. What you're smelling probably isn't being made on the premises. It probably came from miles away in one of those huge container lorries.

23. Shop with a List
You'll save calories and money, too. No impulse buying. And try and shop around the edges of the supermarket. That's where they usually have the fruits, the vegetables, the meats, the dairy products and the bread. Once you're in the aisles, you're in trouble. That's where they keep the biscuits and sweets, the 'convenience' food and junk. Plead fatigue and see if you can get one of the staff to bring you the cereal, then buy all your cleaning stuff and paper supplies at the local shop.

24. Be Suspicious of Food That's Not Where It Should Be
Supermarkets know about merchandising. That's why you're walking along looking for your Diet Pepsi and you come upon the cordial concentrate in a little display carton alongside it. Or you head for your strawberries and you find the pastry cases and whipped cream, nowhere near where

they should be. Supermarkets generally push snack foods – foods that aren't essential or important nutritionally – in this fashion. Notice they don't do it with foods generally regarded as good for you. I've never seen anyone display onions together with the liver.

25. Start Reading the Labels on Food

You look inside your dresses, don't you? You sneak a look under your hostess's plate to see what brand of china she's using. Why aren't you looking to find out what's going into your mouth?

I bought a frozen dessert from a strolling vendor because he told me it was made with skim milk and real fruit. Low-cal, I thought. As I peeled off the wrapper, I noticed that among the ingredients were whipped cream and sugar syrup. And the vendor had such an honest-looking face . . .

Lay off the canned and processed food: it's full of salt and sugar and additives, as you'll know once you read the labels.

You'll come across some other eye-openers. For example, you should know that the ingredients are listed in order: whatever there's most of comes first, whatever there's next most of is second, and so forth. A lot of cleaning products list 'aqueous solution' as the first ingredient. 'Aqueous solution' is just water. Water is also the primary ingredient in a lot of 'fruit' drinks. I wonder how many people realize that 'all-natural' fruit drinks are often 10 per cent fruit, plus water and fructose – it may be natural, because it's not made in a laboratory, but it's sugar.

You should lay off the juices anyway. One ½ pint/300 ml glass is the equivalent of two or more pieces of the real thing. If Nature meant you to get fruit two or three pieces at a time, the serpent would have offered Eve a can and a straw.

26. When You Get the Eating Out of the Closet, Take Your Fat Clothes Along with It

Get rid of those fat clothes. They're just a set-up for failure.

You figure if the diet doesn't work out, your roomy clothes will take you back in. They're your enemy. Give them away. Donate them to the Salvation Army. If you have a lot of weight to lose, I know it's going to be difficult to manage a wardrobe. But you can certainly alter your larger things. Not only will they look better, but you'll be encouraged to keep going. Once a tailor takes out a couple of inches of a dart, there's no going back. Also, buy just a few inexpensive things in your new size – maybe a pair of trousers and two or three blouses. You need and deserve to feel good. At the very least, you can always get a belt for the dresses you just used to let hang. You'll be happy about every new notch.

27. Wear Form-fitting Clothes

My idea of a person who looks good in a tent is Lawrence of Arabia. I've been there. Not to Arabia, but in a lot of those tent dresses. I had enough tent dresses to hold a good-size lawn party underneath them. Now here's the sad truth. Those dresses just make you look heavier. Get out of your 'float'. (I love that euphemism. The dress designers must have had a good laugh choosing it. As everyone knows, a float is a large moving object that belongs in a parade.) Just because you're not wearing a belt, you're not fooling anyone. The opposite may be true: those dresses are an obvious attempt to hide fat.

Start wearing clothes that reveal your body. For one thing, when you try and fit into clothes with zippers and waistlines, you're forced to take a good look at yourself and honestly figure out how much you should lose. In the second place, as your fat starts to disappear, your friends will notice sooner. You deserve to be complimented.

28. Get a Proxy Eater

Society women often show up on the arms of 'walkers' who escort them to parties while their husbands are busy making the bucks. While I recommend you exercise alone, I can see the benefit of a walker to take to parties. While you're at it, get an eater, too. That's a person who comes along with you and eats all the stuff you'd like to but can't. I always get a vicarious thrill from a proxy eater, who is ideally a very thin person with a high metabolic rate.

My friend Joanie is an executive who has to go to a lot of expense account lunches, and she found that some people were uncomfortable when she was dieting and eating 400-calorie lunches, and they were not. She started bringing her assistant Heather along as a proxy eater so her guests wouldn't have to indulge alone. Joanie lost her weight, but Heather, who hadn't been eating expense account lunches till then, ate so much rich food that she worked herself out of her size eights and up to size eighteens. She moved to Hawaii, where she's known as Honolulu Heather, the Muumuu Mama. I'm sending her a copy of the Help Yourself programme.

29. In Restaurants, Don't Read the Menu

It's not as if you're an extraterrestrial. You know your way around a menu. You've been in a restaurant before. You pretty much know what the place is going to have. Make up your mind what you should be eating without looking at the menu – grilled fish, steak, baked chicken, green salad with no dressing, vegetables. Sure there will come a time when you can eat like a thin person, but while you're trying to stay within a calorie limit, you're better off keeping it simple. I'd stay out of ethnic restaurants at the beginning of a diet if I were in your situation – which I have been, of course.

30. Don't Take Any Guff from Waiters

Most waiters and waitresses are pretty good eggs, but every once in a while you run into one of those characters straight out of *Five Easy Pieces* who told Jack Nicholson he couldn't get toast. (Remember what he did? He ordered chicken salad. On white bread: *toasted* white bread. Then, as the waitress headed for the kitchen, he added, 'And hold the chicken salad.')

Don't let yourself be intimidated in restaurants. Just keep telling yourself that in most restaurants, particularly if they have a bar, they've seen everything. Now, I'm not advising, as they do on a certain other diet that's floating around, that you hand the waiter or waitress a little piece of paper with a list of foods you would like, most of which probably aren't on the menu. That's just asking for a cheap crack.

On the other hand, asking to substitute a vegetable for the potato or requesting that your fish be grilled without butter shouldn't get a rude response. I remind you of this because I know that fat people are often shy about asserting themselves in restaurants. They secretly feel everyone is thinking, what are you doing here anyway? You've had enough to eat in your life already.

31. HP Sauce Is the Dieter's Best Friend
Not on steak. On layer cake. If you're tempted to nibble when you've had enough, or when there's something on the plate that you absolutely should not eat, put HP sauce over it. Of course I understand that for lunch President Ford topped his cottage cheese with HP because he actually preferred it that way, but for me, putting HP sauce on anything but meat is the kiss of death. Alternative: pour on the salt. It may not be the suavest move you'll ever make in a restaurant, but who cares?

32. Start Learning About Nutrition
Even though I'd like to, I can't cram everything you should know about the subject between the covers of this book. There are libraries full of information. You'll be improving your mind along with your body, and you'll have something to talk about at cocktail parties instead of circling around the buffet. Just be careful that with all your new-found information you don't make the hostess feel too guilty about serving all the liquor and the hors d'oeuvres

laced with monosodium glutamate that cause brain damage.

33. Don't Serve Meals in Serving Platters
Serve yourself and your family in the kitchen – or near the stove if you eat in the kitchen – giving everyone the appropriate amount. Avoid the temptation of having a heaped bowlful of anything right in front of your dinner plate. If your family wants seconds, let them go back into the kitchen for them. The walk will probably do them good.

34. Discuss Food or Dieting Only While You're Eating
Did you ever notice that slim people unselfconsciously discuss what they're eating, while fat people discuss what they're not eating? ('I only had half a carton of cottage cheese all day.' Of course, sometimes they lie.) Both subjects are relatively boring once you've left the dining-room and therefore should not be discussed unless you're a member of a culinary society, which I would definitely not advise. Take up another hobby, like skin-diving. It's hard to snack under water.

35. When It's Over, It's Over
'Tomorrow' should be your new theme song. There's always tomorrow to start eating some more. When you've finished a meal, put your fork down and get away from the table – fast. Clear the dishes off, and get out of the room. Preferably you'll get right out of the house and take a moderate walk.

36. Don't Hang Around the Kitchen
Get out of there. If you're in the kitchen, I'd bet it's not to admire the wallpaper. Allow yourself a run-through only. The less time you spend surrounded by food and food accessories the better. This goes not only for your kitchen, but other people's. Sit in the garden; sit in the living-room. Don't even offer to help clean up at parties. Let other people do it for a change.

37. Rehearse High-Risk Situations

When I was anticipating a special occasion, I used to think beforehand about what I was going to eat. I still do, only now it takes me a lot less time because there's a lot less I plan to eat. I actually try and picture myself in a situation that I know will be difficult – a party, a holiday dinner, a meal in a favourite restaurant – and I decide very specifically what I will do. If I've decided I'll have two drinks, I follow a plan and drink them on schedule. Otherwise, I might conveniently 'forget' how many I've had and go overboard. It's also very easy to overeat when friends urge you to join them, unless you've decided ahead of time that you will stay in control and made up your mind how.

38. Keep Those Emergency Stores Out of the House

I once calculated that if three dozen refugees landed on my doorstep in the middle of the night, I could serve them four butter shortbread fingers apiece. If they didn't land, I had plenty for myself. I didn't even have to go through the trouble of baking them. I could just eat them right from the pack.

I had a friend who really loved birthday cake. He'd go around town ordering cakes – 'Happy Birthday, Barry,' 'Happy Birthday, Brad,' and so forth – then go home and eat them by himself. He started freezing the cakes, so he wouldn't eat them all at once. Then he discovered that the best place for food to thaw is in your stomach.

Anything fattening that's lying around the house, I discovered, soon wound up in my mouth. While you still haven't got control of your eating, keep it out. I read some diet tips about storing the fattening food out of sight, in the back of the cabinet. What I want to know is what it's doing there in the first place. If you're worried about your friends coming over and finding the cupboard bare, maybe this is a good time to think about who your friends are, anyway. Are they coming for your companionship . . . or your cake? More important: are you keeping the stuff for them . . . or for yourself?

39. When the Guests Leave, the Party's Over

I think a really pathetic sight is a guy wearing a party hat standing in an empty room, in the middle of a pile of dirty plates, stuffing his face with the leftovers. Once your friends have gone home, throw away everything that hasn't been eaten. If you can't bear to do that, wrap up the food and send it home with your guests as if it were wedding cake. Tell them they'll be doing you a big favour by getting it out of the house. Otherwise, the leftover will turn into a hangover – the kind that hangs over your belt.

40. Find a New Hangout

As a rule of thumb, stay away from any place where the waitress says to you, 'Can I bring you the usual?' If I know you, the usual is not a watercress sandwich. Certain places trigger certain kinds of behaviour. If your hangout is the local pub, you're going to be awfully tempted to order your favourite cocktail; or maybe your weakness is the apple pie at the take-away. Stay away until you're really in control.

41. Don't Join a Fancy Health Club

As if it isn't discouraging enough to have to sign those releases absolving blame if the programme sends you out of the door feet first, you also have to cope with the instructors. Those same people who chose you last for their teams in high school are now supposed to be helping you get into shape, and it's been my experience they're about as sympathetic and helpful as Miss Hannigan was to Little Orphan Annie. I have always felt that fancy health clubs are really just places where people obsessed with their bodies can show them off when it isn't nice enough to go to the beach.

42. Avoid Diet Schemes

If somebody you met at a party tried to get you to back the Society of Levitationists, you'd think he was crazy. Then how come when Cousin Suzie comes for the weekend with another of her loony diets you go over the moon? You start taking notes about some wild programme that involves watermelon and horseradish and you're ready to start following it like the Holy Grail.

You know that song 'My Way'? I think it should be the theme song for dieters. Everybody's got another method that's going to get those twenty pounds off you fast and forever. One thing I can assure you: if it happens fast, it won't be forever.

Do yourself a favour. You've already spent the money on this book. Follow the programme. It's going to work. Then when you next see Cousin Suzie, if she hasn't already gone to her Great Reward in the Sky from the botulism in her diet protein shake, you can lend her this book so she can start losing the weight she's gained since last year.

43. Remember That a Diet Is Not a Punishment
It's not great having to write down all your calories and keep exercising. But consider the alternatives. Do you enjoy living in bed and having your view of your toes blocked by your stomach? Lying down is a good place to examine how overweight you truly are, since in that position your fat is generally distributed as evenly as possible. I knew I was in trouble when I couldn't locate my hipbones when I was flat on my back. Don't be annoyed that you're on a diet. Remember you had a pretty good time before you started. Now try telling yourself that a diet is not something you're *enduring*, it's something you're *doing*. Be proud of yourself and think how great it will be to live like a lean and fit person.

44. Don't Believe Your Mother
That very same woman who told you that there was a Santa Claus, that the stork brought babies, and that you were prettier than any Miss America is now telling you that you look too thin. Don't believe her. Unfortunately, well-meaning mums, along with loving friends and devoted spouses, have a hard time accepting a fitter you when they're

used to a fatter you. Give them some time to get used to the new way you look. It is possible to diet to excess, but if you follow the Help Yourself programme – particularly the part about adding calories – you will be eating properly and you will be at a weight that is appropriate and healthy for you.

Part Three
Second Helpings

Second Helpings are for people who haven't had enough. I'm hoping that includes you. It includes me: at this point in the book I still haven't had a chance to share all the things I've discovered about food, nutrition, and exercise. That's why I've added this section.

Some of the questions in Q&A are ones I myself asked Dr Joel. Fiction/Fact includes some of my favourite (wrong) notions that I've now been corrected on. Did You Know That? . . . is full of facts you should know, and Other Ways to Fry a Fish, which is not about frying fish, is full of cooking suggestions I think you'll find useful. And that's just a part of what Second Helpings is about.

Nibbles comes first, because for dieters, nibbles have to go first! I know it seems hard: when I first swore off buttered muffins, I wondered what would get me out of bed in the morning! I don't get my kicks from fat-rich goodies any more. I get them from feeling great about myself.

14. Nibbles

Do you think about food too much? Try this word association test and find out.

Tonsillectomy	a) Operation	b) Ice cream
Picnic	a) Ants	b) Pork pie
Weddings	a) Brides	b) Cake
Ronald Reagan	a) President	b) Jelly beans
Romance	a) Valentines	b) Chocolates
Circus	a) Clown	b) Custard pie
Virility	a) Warren Beatty	b) Oysters
Mum	a) Pop	b) Cake-baking
Pop	a) Mum	b) Glass of beer
Illness	a) Doctors	b) Chicken soup

The World's Most Fattening Beverage Eggnog has 335 calories per four-ounce serving.

The Pilgrim Fathers got their first taste of popcorn in America at the first Thanksgiving dinner – which, by the way, was really a breakfast served by Indian chief Massasoit's brother to the Pilgrims and ninety-two members of his tribe. Dessert was popcorn, which I believe everyone ate plain. So should you. Here's why:

Popcorn, 8 oz/225 g dry: 40 calories
Popcorn, 8 oz/225 g popped with fat and salt: 81 calories
Popcorn, 8 oz/225 g popped with a sugar coating: 134 calories

At a ½ teaspoon per stick, 60 per cent of a stick of chewing gum is pure sugar. Nineteen per cent is cornflour. One stick of gum has about 9 calories. Sugarless chewing gum has about 8 calories per stick.

A few brands of sugarless chewing gum are sweetened with 'aspartame' – a sweetener that's about twenty-one times as potent as sugar. Four calories' worth of aspartame, though, is as sweet as two teaspoons of sugar (36 calories). So far, it hasn't been okayed for use in soft drinks, but it can appear in cold breakfast cereals, puddings, dessert toppings and other products.

The party's over . . . before the main course, if you hit the hors d'oeuvres. A strolling snacker can take in as many calories as if she's eaten a full-course meal. Check the chart below before you run for the cocktail plate:

Item	Calories
3 Cheddars or 2 rye crispbreads	63
with	
1 oz/25 g Cheddar cheese (enough for 3 crackers)	112
2 chicken livers wrapped in bacon	180
1 fried chicken wing	54
2 medium frankfurters	78
½ Butter Puff	27
with	
1 oz/25 g chicken liver pâté	80
10 peanuts	105
	689

It may be a once-a-year thing, but the party's still over . . . if you nibble on these 'occasional' foods. Maybe it's a birthday, a company bash, an engagement party. The merrymaker may make herself miserable the next day just remembering how she celebrated a happy event. Check the figures below before you lift a forkful:

Item	Calories
8 fl oz/225 ml champagne	164
1 oz/25 g Brie cheese with	94
1 Cornish Wafer	45
1 oz/ 25 g cream crackers	158
3 spareribs with barbecue sauce	168
1 serving of vanilla ice cream with	145
1 piece of butter sponge with chocolate icing	163
	937

Blame the Swiss Milk chocolate was first made in Switzerland in 1876.

The Reverend Sylvester W. Graham (for whom the Graham cracker was named) was one-time preacher and food faddist who believed that pepper, mustard and ketchup caused insanity.

I wouldn't go that far. Pepper's a respectable spice. In fact, hot red pepper has more vitamin C per oz/25 g than any other fruit or vegetable. (Only the Human Torch could knock back that much of the fiery stuff.) Although a sprinkling of black pepper doesn't boast a high vitamin content, it does add snap to foods, with barely any calories. Mustard is actually a blend of mustard seed or powder, flour, and other spices in a base of either water, wine, vinegar or champagne. Mustard has about 4 calories per teaspoon. Ketchup averages about 20 calories per tablespoon, depending on the brand, not because of the main ingredient (tomatoes), but because of the sugar content. Some ketchups are about one-third to one-quarter sugar.

America's favourite side order is french fried potatoes. Ten fries, about 2×½×½ inch/5×1×1 cm, have 156 calories. Who eats just ten?

Second Helpings

Ga-ga over goobers The average American consumes about 3½ lb/1.4 kg peanut butter a year. In fact, I suspect that most people eat none, while all the rest is consumed by kids and the mums who make their sandwiches. Three tablespoons of peanut butter have 288 calories and 23.9 grams of fat.

Peanuts are nutritious, but fattening. ¾ oz/20 g salted peanuts gives you 105 calories and 10.7 grams of fat – about a quarter of a day's allowance. Sugar plus nuts are a caloric double whammy: peanut brittle has 128 calories per 1 oz/25 g piece. Don't go nuts with nuts.

You have 9000 taste buds on your tongue. Nature was very clever in placing them: the tip determines sweetness, the sides, salt. The taste buds for picking up sourness are located farther back on the sides; bitterness is picked up way back on your tongue. These are the four basic tastes with shades between them.

Before it's on the tip of your tongue, reconsider your breakfast order: do you really want that porridge with cream and sugar (270 calories)?

I hate to admit this, but . . . pizza is not just 'empty calories'. It's a pretty nutritious nibble. Experts say it's fairly well-balanced for fast food, with protein, carbohydrates, fat, vitamin A and some minerals. Still, one 17-calorie slice is about 27 per cent fat.

The thicker the crust and the more pepperoni and/or anchovies are laid on, the more the calories and fat content go up. Pizza is an okay *snack* for a growing teenager to eat. Pizza, for you and me, is a *meal*.

Speaking of fast food: I didn't grow up with fast food joints, take-aways and mobile ice cream stalls lying in wait on every corner the way they are today, and you probably didn't either.

Fast food places are great once in a while, more as a matter of convenience than as 'restaurants' that serve balanced meals. The food you get in fast food shops is high in protein, but also high in fat and salt – and if you go for the straw-clogging thick milkshakes, high in sugar, too.

Fast food menus are low (or lacking) in fresh fruit dishes and cooked vegetables. Don't expect to find low-cal nibbles. Even a dish that sounds as if it might be for a dieter, like 'Chef's Special Fresh Salad Platter', can have 800 calories, nearly twice as much as a 7-oz/200-g Findus cheese and tomato pizza.

Fourteen reasons to nibble and/or binge you should never use again:

You're worried
It's that time of month
You're lonely
You've just had a fight
You can always diet
You're frustrated
You're bored
You're nervous

You don't want to waste food others have left over
You're going through a crisis
It's 'health' food so it's good for you
You need a pep up
You're happy
It's there

Dubious designer binge When asked by *Cosmopolitan*, 'What do you do when you go on a binge?' Gloria Vanderbilt replied: 'Cinnamon on cottage cheese. I pretend it's rice pudding.'

The fourth biggest lie One size fits all.

15. Q&A

What's the difference between low-cal and reduced calorie foods? How can you tell which fish is fattiest before biting into it? Answers to these questions and others you've wondered about follow . . .

Q: Help! I loved the diets that let you eat all the meat you wanted. Now you tell me to eat only 5 oz/150 g steak. That isn't much.

A: An 8 oz/225 g T-bone steak, grilled, has 545 calories. Not good. Worse yet, it seems that a diet high in fat and protein may pose a greater risk of cancer than cigarette smoking. The word comes from a Cornell University nutritionist.

A typical American gets 40–60 per cent of his calories from fats. Ideally, so a government Committee on Nutrition and Human Needs has found, the typical American should get 50–65 per cent from carbohydrates, 15–20 per cent from protein, and 20–30 per cent from fats. Studies show that fat intake exceeding 35 per cent of total calories is associated with cancers of the colon, prostate, breast and large bowel. Diet may be the most important risk factor for cancer.

The diet recommended to decrease the risk of cancer is the same one that has been associated with a decreased likelihood of cardiovascular disease and diabetes.

This should discourage you from making meat the mainstay of your diet – whether or not you're trying to cut calories. You're eating meat out of habit, and you need to re-educate yourself to control the food. The food shouldn't control you.

Q: Okay. Now that I know about limiting my intake of beef, won't I be spending more to buy the cheaper cuts? Don't good cuts have less fat than the cheaper ones?

A: Not at all. It depends which part of the animal the meat comes from. Lean minced beef, generally made from less good cuts and trimmings, is kept if possible to no more than 25 per cent fat.

Even so, a lot of fat melts out when you cook a hamburger. Grill it so fat drips off into the pan below.

Extra lean beef with about 15–20 per cent fat is your best buy. You lose less volume because of fat melting out and end up with more lean beef.

If you're preparing beef for the family, choose topside, rump or thick flank for roasting. These are usually leaner than sirloin, forerib or rolled ribs.

Q: Is all fish low in calories?

A: Fish is not only categorized by whether it's fresh or salt-water bred, but also (among other qualities) by size, shape and fat content. Generally, you can spot the fattier fish in a flash – the darker the flesh, the higher the fat content.

A fattier-fleshed fish is better suited to grilling or roasting because of the extra oil in it. A leaner-fleshed fish is generally cooked in oil or butter – which may bring the calorie count up to more than a same-sized serving of a fattier cousin. Instead, grill or steam it.

Here are a few example of fatty v. less fatty fish per 3½ oz/85 g serving, uncooked, based on statistics from the United States Department of Agriculture:

Atlantic salmon: 217 calories   Atlantic and Pacific halibut:
Rainbow trout: 195 calories   100 calories
Pacific mackerel: 159 calories Cod: 78 calories
Tuna: 145 calories   Haddock: 75 calories
Striped bass: 105 calories   Coley: 75 calories
Whiting: 105 calories

Here's a piece of information to drop at dinner parties: the tail end of the fish has a stronger flavour because of the exercise the fish gets from swimming around, but the tail meat's a bit less tender than the rest.

Q: I've seen tofu at health food shops. What is it?
A: Tofu is a low-calorie, fairly nutritious soybean cake that's a good, inexpensive vegetable protein source. Tofu is made by mashing soybeans into soymilk, then pressing the curd mixture into a solid cake. Tofu has about 9.4 grams of protein in a 2 inch/5 cm square, no cholesterol, minimal saturated fat, and 72 calories per 3½ oz/ 85 g.

They are available in long-life cartons in most health food shops and are inexpensive as protein foods go.

Q: What's the difference between 'reduced calorie' food and 'low calorie' foods?
A: When a food is labelled 'reduced calories', you will find it has one-third fewer calories per serving than a comparable food made by another company. If a food is labelled 'low calorie', you should get no more than 40 calories per serving.

Q: Aren't pasta, potatoes, and bread no-nos on a diet?
A: You've been scared off from all carbohydrates – wrongly. Carbohydrates come in two forms. One is simple sugars, which are absorbed right into your system with a minimal amount of processing to give you instant energy. When instant energy supplies run out, you still need energy.

You get it from the other form of carbohydrates: starches. They are just complex sugars that take longer to process than simple sugars. The breakdown of starch helps keep you from feeling fatigued. If your body is short of carbohydrates, it will begin to break down muscle (protein) to make simple sugars. *This* is a no-no.

Q: Aren't condensed milk and evaporated milk the same?
A: No more than malted milk and skim milk! A tablespoon

of condensed milk has 64 calories, thanks to the added sugar. Evaporated has 22, whole milk (3.25 per cent fat) has 11, and skim has 5 per tablespoon. Some people think evaporated skim milk tastes 'richer' in coffee than skim and gives the coffee a better colour. Try it.

Q: Can I eat sugarless mints and chewing gum?
A: You're supposed to break the habit of eating – or having something in your mouth – between meals. Besides, some folks suffer wind attacks from 'sugarless' mints or gum that contains xylitol or sorbitol. If you blame that slightly bloated feeling on whatever you ate before you popped in a mint, think again.

Cause of the wind? We can't digest certain carbohydrates. When they hit the intestines, bacteria that live there ferment the undigested stuff and, bingo – wind. Beans have the dubious honour of creating the most of this stuff. Other culprits: cabbage, spinach, grapes, cereal bran and even innocent-seeming apple juice.

Q: If I exercise an hour every day, do I have to cut calories, too?
A: Farrah Fawcett once said that since she exercises so much, she eats all she wants. If you follow the plan, some day you too will be able to eat like Farrah, though I can't guarantee you'll *look* like her. If you're just starting the programme, let me remind you that exercising without cutting calorie intake *will* eventually lead to a weight loss. The key word is *eventually*. No dieter I know was ever interested in *slow* weight loss. So cut your calories while you exercise and you'll get to your goal that much quicker.

Q: How long do I need to exercise before I know I'm burning body fat, not just losing water by perspiring?
A: Obviously, when you exercise strenuously you begin to perspire. The reason you sweat during exercise is the same reason you sweat when the weather's hot – it's your body's

187

way of cooling you down. After about fifteen minutes of exercise, if you really work at it, you begin to perspire. After half an hour to forty-five minutes, you are using body fat for energy and fuel.

In case you wondered: the average woman's brain weighs forty-four ounces; the average man's, forty-nine ounces. When you're not exercising, your brain uses 66 per cent of the glucose in your body, while your muscles divide up the rest. Your less-than-three-pound brain uses up as much glucose as some thirty-to-seventy pounds of muscle (depending on your body size).

16. Fact/Fiction

There's an old superstition that thunderstorms curdle milk. This is only true if the storm causes power failure and your refrigerator, with milk in it, shuts off. Other myths about food (and your body) need some clearing up, too.

Fiction Grapefruit and pineapple will burn body fat.
Fact Over the years, grapefruit has been the main ingredient in several 'miracle' reducing plans. It's a fine food, with few calories and plenty of vitamin C, but it doesn't burn body fat. Same for pineapple. No such fat-burning food has yet been discovered. When it is, I'm buying it all.

Fiction Brown rice and enriched rice have the same nutritional value, while wild rice has more calories.
Fact Brown rice is parboiled and heat-treated before it is dried, milled, and packaged. Heat treating draws the nutrients from the rice bran and germ into the grain. When white rice is processed, the bran and germ are removed. White rice then may be 'enriched' with some nutrients (after being stripped of them), but it's not as nutritious as brown rice. It's also higher in calories.

Fiction Bananas are fattening.
Fact Compared to apples and oranges, the banana is sweeter: a ripe banana is about 21 per cent sugar, an apple 14 per cent sugar and an orange 12 per cent. Yet the average 3½-ounce (6-inch) banana has only 85 calories. A medium apple has 80 calories and an orange has 80 calories.

That 3½-ounce banana has 1.1 grams of protein and plenty

of potassium, but no cholesterol – good for healthy hearts. Bananas also have a very mild laxative effect – the fibre and pectin in the fruit purportedly aid in curbing constipation. It takes your system three hours to digest a banana.

In case you wondered if there were any banana-holics around, the answer's yes. Natives of Buganda, Uganda are bananas over bananas. According to *The Total Banana* by Alex Abella, the average Bugandan consumes about nine pounds of bananas per day – that's about 2½ bananas per waking hour.

Fiction 'Sugar-free' foods have fewer calories than those with sugar.
Fact No such luck. 'Sugar free' only means that there's no sugar in the product – the manufacturer wasn't pulling your leg on that. However, it doesn't mean that what you're buying isn't loaded with other sweeteners which have as many calories or *more* than sugar. Ice creams or desserts flavoured with honey may have more calories because honey has more calories per teaspoon than sugar. Corn syrup, fructose, sorbitol and molasses are other high-calorie additions. When you buy something that says it's sugar free, compare the calorie count to a similar product made with sugar. Of course, the sweetest reward comes from being able to pass the stuff by, sugar free or not.

Fiction There are fewer calories in 1 lb/450 g soft tub margarine than in the non-whipped block or tub varieties.
Fact There are fewer calories in the soft tub stuff *only if you use less of it.* 1 lb/450 g soft tub margarine has the same calorie count as 1 lb/450 g block margarine.

Soft tub margarine has been processed to prevent it hardening, that's all, so you can spread it more thinly. The smaller the serving, the fewer the calories.

Fiction Margarine has fewer calories than butter.
Fact By law, both butter and margarine must have the same

fat content (80 per cent milk fat). However, most margarines have little if any cholesterol since they consist mostly of unsaturated fats such as vegetable oils.

Here's the catch. Unsaturated vegetable oils become somewhat saturated when they have been processed to make them solid. You wind up with 100 calories per tablespoon for both butter and margarine.

Low-cal butter-type spreads such as Outline or Gold contain less fat and more water and therefore have fewer calories. Outline has half the calories of butter and margarine.

Fiction Foods like celery and apples have 'negative calories' because of the energy needed to chew and digest them.

Fact A calorie is a calorie is a calorie, whether you're eating apples or strawberry shortcake. An average-size person uses only 0.3 calories per minute while eating. That means a 5-calorie stalk of celery would have to be chewed for seventeen minutes to have no caloric value. I imagine you have better things to do.

Fiction Aubergine is a meat substitute.

Fact Only by reputation. Like most vegetables, aubergine is mostly water. In fact, it's 93 per cent water. Four per cent of this vegetable is carbohydrate.

Aubergine is probably thought of as a meat substitute because it's commonly used in popular dishes like meat. This vegetable has certain physical qualities that make it practical to use in such recipes. It can be sliced into 'steaks', breaded and fried without falling apart – under a watchful eye. It also works like a blotter – it soaks up cooking oil as it loses its water content when in the pan.

4 oz/100 g aubergine, cooked with no oil, has only 38 calories and about 2 grams of protein. Add breadcrumbs, cheese, and fry in oil, and the calorie count and fat content soar. Don't blame it on the aubergine.

Fiction Your stomach shrinks as you diet.
Fact When you diet successfully, you become accustomed to eating less food. Your stomach is the same size as always.

Fiction Using 'non-dairy' cream substitutes or dessert toppings saves calories.
Fact Sorry. Non-dairy creams have more calories per tablespoon than milk since most of them are made with coconut oil. Coconut has the highest saturated fat content per gram of any other vegetable oil. Coffee-mate has 21.7 per cent saturated fats and 11 calories per teaspoon. Many dessert toppings are made from coconut oil, too.

Fiction Lecithin pills burn fat.
Fact Sorry, not a chance. Lecithin is a fat. Your body reacts to commercially made lecithin pills as it would to other fats: it breaks it down and sends it through your system. Here's the surprise: lecithin pills have calories – in fact, 9 calories per pill.

17. Did You Know That? . . .

Thomas Jefferson, America's third President, was responsible for importing to America rice, the waffle iron, Calcutta hogs, Neapolitan macaroni, French wines, french fries, ice cream, mustard, Parmesan cheese, vanilla, olive oil, asparagus, and broccoli. Other facts about food, fat and exercise may be just as surprising to you. For example, did you know that:

● White meat roasted turkey and dark meat roasted chicken have the same calorie count (176 calories per 3½ oz/ 85 g), but dark meat turkey is about 40 per cent fattier.

● Artichokes, rich in potassium and iron, have only 44 calories per cooked globe (base and soft ends of the leaves). If you just like the hearts, skip the ones swimming in jars of oil, and head for the kind canned in brine. Artichoke hearts without oil have only 26 calories per 3½ oz/85 g! Add a few to a salad. Another plus: one artichoke contains four times the fibre of a bran scone.

● Tuna in brine has about 20 per cent more protein and up to 161 fewer calories per 3½-oz/85-g serving than oil-packed. Brine-packed tuna is about 99 per cent protein and 1 per cent fat. Tuna gives you three to four times the niacin (which helps break down starch and sugar, so important in dieting) and one-fourth more vitamin B_{12} (which helps your blood cells carry oxygen, important in exercising) than steak.

● Cooking sherry of the supermarket variety contains

about one teaspoon of salt per 8 fl oz/225 ml, plus other flavourings, and the calorie count is 76.

● Dry roasted peanuts have just about the same amount of calories as cocktail peanuts cooked in oil. A lot.

● If you use plain low-fat yogurt instead of sour cream, you save about 273 calories per 8 fl oz/225 ml.

● Lean roasted beef topside has fewer calories and a lower fat count than lean roasted leg of lamb. Two slices of lamb: 107 calories and 3.5 grams of fat. Two slices of topside: 78 calories and 1.1 grams of fat.

● You may think you're saving tons of calories by eating a sorbet instead of ice cream; you're not. You do get less fat in a sorbet but you'll also be getting more sugar. 4 fl oz/120 ml sorbet equals 120–150 calories, depending on the flavour and the brand.

● At 61 calories a tablespoon, honey has more calories than sugar (46 calories a tablespoon).

● Except for unsalted or low-salt cottage cheese or any cheese made especially low in salt, *all* cheeses are high in sodium. How did the salt get in? Not only are salt and other sodium compounds added for flavour, they're also used to control acidity and curb undesirable bacterial growth. Some pasteurized processed cheeses are very high in sodium – up to 490 milligrams per 1 oz/25 g. (See chapter 18 for more on salt.)

● Vegetables that are steamed are more nutritious than vegetables cooked in water. It takes longer, though: steam doesn't conduct heat as well as boiling water. As usual, patience is a virtue: you'll get more out of steamed vegetables.

● There's about 6 per cent more sugar in frozen yogurt than in standard commercial ice cream.

● Imported Brie cheese has about a 50 per cent fat content. Supposedly, Brie sold in France has only a 40 per cent fat content. This is not a Gallic plot: it's just that pasteurized milk is used in the exported product.

● Clarified stock and consommé are not strictly the same thing, though they have identical calorie counts. Clarified stock is a clear or almost clear soup that's usually lightly seasoned. Consommé, too, is a clear soup, but is much stronger and is more heavily seasoned. Clarified beef stock and consommé have 23 calories per 8 fl oz/225 ml; chicken 22 calories per 8 fl oz/225 ml. Go easy on commercially made soups like these: they tend to be on the salty side.

● Milk and other dairy products aren't the only good sources of calcium. Cabbage, broccoli and kale are also rich sources. Calcium is especially important to women approaching middle age, when they're candidates for the bone disorder osteoporosis.

● Pistachio nuts have 88 calories per 30 nuts. Cashews come in at 280 calories for between 20–26 nuts.

● When you see the words 'non-nutritive crude fibre' listed in your cereal's ingredients, you're paying extra for, yes, *wood* fibre. Crude fibre won't make you sick, but neither do you need it. Fibre from grain and fruits, though, are another story. An increase in fibre is recommended by many doctors – fibre has been shown to regulate bowels and may decrease the risk of colon cancer.

● 10½ small water biscuits (at 14 calories each) have the same calorie count as a scoop of chocolate ice cream (147 calories).

● Though you might have been taught that vegetables that are yellow or reddish are high in vitamin A, it's not so with beetroot and radishes. One large carrot has 650 times as much vitamin A as two raw medium-sized beetroot and 11,000 times the vitamin A in ten radishes. Beetroot is also low in protein, vitamin C and iron. For 43 calories (two beetroot), you get mostly flavour and a great colour. However . . . beetroot tops are great. They are high in vitamin A, a good source of calcium and provide one-third of your RDA of iron. Radishes are pretty low in nutrients – they have only that snappy taste and low-calorie count going for them. Ten have 17 calories.

● Smaller hens, turkeys and chickens are leaner than the larger ones.

● Depending on the type of mix you use (homemade or commercial), just under two-thirds or so of the calories (260–290) in an average slice of fruit-filled pie come from the top and bottom crusts alone. And you know why. The crust is flour, water and fat – and of course, some sugar.

● Two 12-oz/350-ml cans of beer amount to 320 calories. That's nearly *one-third* of a dieter's daily calorie intake.

● A hot dog roll has 108 calories, a hamburger bun, 89. A typical hot dog weighs 1¾ oz/45 g and has 124 calories; a 3 oz/75 g burger (about the size you get at a fast food place) has 140. You get more meat, less nitrites, and about the same calories when you choose a small hamburger rather than a hot dog. Watch out for those giant burgers, though – they're calorie-loaded.

● 1 oz/25 g cheddar cheese has 122 calories. If you always thought hard cheeses were a good source of protein, you were wrong. Only about 25 per cent of the calories are protein. The rest are fat.

● Turkey yields more edible protein, minus fat or skin, than chicken or duck. You'll get about 46 per cent protein with turkey, 41 per cent with chicken and 22 per cent for ducklings. (Another reason not to wait for Christmas.)

● Not all processed cheeses are made entirely of cheese. Government regulations lay down how much real cheese each type must contain. The kind sold in slices or small portions is generally just called processed cheese and it contains more real cheese than the softer spreadable kinds called cheese spreads. Both also contain emulsifiers, water, salt, colouring and spices or flavourings. Most processed cheese slices and portions sold in Britain have between 93 and 104 calories per 1 oz/25 g. Cheese spreads have between 73 and 83 calories per 1 oz/25 g.

● You have a slimmer chance of being on TV if you're heavy. John J. O'Connor in *The New York Times* noted that while in the real world, 'a substantial' number of people are overweight, 'the tube world' shows a different picture. A 1979 study revealed that on television, only 2 per cent of women and 6 per cent of men were fat.

● Those vibrating belt machines are about as effective in melting away fat as a girdle is. You have to work muscle and expend energy to lose body fat. You can't lose fat while the machine shakes you up. You're the one who should be moving – not the machine.

● No comment: 'There are certain compensations for overweight women. Men do not suspect them and other women do not fear them as competition.' Elsa Maxwell, in her autobiography, *RSVP*.

18. The Most Dangerous Things to Put in Your Mouth

Butter

Hey, I know what you're thinking. Everyone knows that butter is dangerous for dieters. Most of us just don't realize how dangerous: 100 calories per tablespoon, and it's a saturated fat. (More on this on the next page.) That calorie count is over twice as high as sugar, over three times as high as bread, ten times as high as potatoes.

A very high calorie count alone is not enough reason to put a food on the top of the danger list. Take cream cheese, for example. The truth is that cream cheese doesn't turn up as often as butter, which goes with almost everything.

I didn't realize how much butter I was eating until my husband decided to total it up. He put a fresh block on the butter dish before breakfast. Well, I'd put a dab on my diet toast. (Of course, I was dieting at the time.) I used a little on my vegetables and a little more on the fish I grilled. By bedtime, I had used 2½ oz/70 g. That was 530 hidden calories. My daily intake on my 1200-calorie-a-day diet had gone up to 1730.

Helpful Hints
- Butter the smooth side of Ryvita Rye Crisp and you'll use half the calories.
- Use softened margarine or butter. It spreads evenly, so you use less.
- Always cool toast before you butter it. Otherwise, the butter will melt into the bread and tempt you to pile on more.
- Whip your butter to make it go further, or seem to.

Fats

Butter has its own category because it's one of the foods that's easy to overdo. Butter's just a fat, and there are other fats we eat with similar abandon – like nuts, ham, cream and cream sauces. Fats are also found in meat, poultry skin, dairy products, non-dairy cream substitutes, margarines and salad oils (which are nothing but). We consume about seven tablespoons of fat a day, but the surprise is we only need one tablespoon's worth to maintain good health.

Without some fat, we'd be in sad trouble. You need fat to help keep a sex-hormone balance, and your skin needs it so it won't dry out. Without fat, you couldn't absorb the fat-soluble vitamins like A, E, D and K.

Fat itself isn't bad, but your fat intake needs watching, specifically fat intake of the wrong sort. Some fats are good guys and some are bad guys.

Saturated fats are the bad guys. A trick to spot them: they're solid at room temperature. Beef fat is one example. In the vegetable kingdom, where most are not saturated, coconut and palm kernel oils are the exceptions. (You'll find these two vegetable fats in some cookies, cakes, non-dairy 'creams' and soured cream, as well as dessert toppings.)

Polyunsaturated fats and oils are usually liquid and are mostly vegetable in origin. Corn, sunflower, walnut, sesame seed, cottonseed and soybean oils are high in polyunsaturated fats. These are the good guys.

Monosaturated fats, the fence-sitters, are considered neither good nor bad. Olive and groundnut oils are monosaturated.

Fats are important to know about for two reasons. They are the most caloric food (9 calories) per gram, and in saturated form, too much can raise your blood cholesterol level. (More on this very soon.)

If you're really into fat follies, you eat fats because they taste good and fill you up. They sneak in all over the place, into every meal. Eat 1 oz/25 g bacon fat and you've taken in 126 calories. 1 oz/25 g pork fat has 216 calories. If you wouldn't touch organ meat (like liver) but are crazy for pâté, guess what: eat pâté and you're eating a variety of fat-laden ingredients including chicken or pork livers plus pork meat, cream, egg yolks, flour, brandy and (often) nuts. The only low-calorie ingredients are the spices. This is why one tablespoon of pâté contains 69 calories (and up) and about 6 grams of fat.

And if you think you're being smart by having half an avocado instead of a fattening meat dinner, you'll not only be eating a food that's 75 per cent fat, but adding about 170 calories to your daily intake.

Helpful Hints
- Limit your intake of fried foods or cut them out entirely.
- Avoid cheese dressings on salads. Sprinkle them with lemon juice and spices instead.
- Avoid creamed soups.
- Steam, grill or poach fish and poultry. Avoid duck or goose, which are very fatty birds. Do not eat poultry skin.
- Trim the fat off meats and buy the leaner cuts.
- Invest in a few non-stick pots and pans. If what you're cooking requires some oil, add a mere drop of a polyunsaturated oil.
- Cut back or avoid nuts (like peanuts) and chocolate syrup, which has saturated fats in it.
- Use low-fat soft cheeses (usually about 4 per cent fat in them) and low-fat dairy products like skim milk, low-fat yogurt, and buttermilk.

Cholesterol
What is this thing called cholesterol and why do we hear so much about it? Cholesterol is critical to life, that's why. We do not have to eat cholesterol-packed foods for our bodies to make use of it – the liver churns out about 1000 milligrams of it a day on its own. Cholesterol stengthens cell membranes and helps manufacture sex hormones, among its other functions. Your liver won't over-produce it, but if *you*

overeat the foods that are jam-packed with the stuff, you have problems.

Scientific evidence points to saturated fats and cholesterol as key culprits in heart and blood vessel diseases. Blocked blood vessels are something you do not want. Supposedly, saturated fats increase the amount of cholesterol in the blood, while polyunsaturates reduce the amount. (Monosaturates have no effect.)

Cholesterol has to get carried through the body some way and 'lipoproteins' do it. There are low-density lipoproteins (LDLs), very-low-density lipoproteins (VLDLs), and high-density lipoproteins (HDLs).

Low-density lipoproteins and very-low-density lipoproteins keep cholesterol circulating around your body. Though the bloodstream has 'scavenger cells' that get rid of some extra cholesterol, in the course of travel, lots of cholesterol manages to attach itself to arteries – and they clog.

To solve this, you want high-density lipoproteins. These HDLs (*which are increased in number by strenuous exercise*) snatch cholesterol from artery walls and ship them back to the liver. The liver doesn't want any excess and excretes the extra cholesterol as bile through the intestines.

Which foods are high in cholesterol? Eggs have the highest concentration per gram of any food. It's also in meats, whole milk, organ meats, and high in some fish like sardines and prawns.

Helpful Hints
- The American Heart Association recommends a cholesterol intake of about 300 milligrams or less a day. Invest in a cholesterol counter and check to see how much you're getting.
- Limit your intake of eggs and foods containing eggs. Three eggs a week should do it.
- Look for hidden eggs in packaged goods and don't discount what you're mixing in batters: they're in cakes, frostings, mayonnaise, noodles, soufflés, waffles,

> hamburger mix, custard, hollandaise sauce, fritters, pancakes and even some pretzels.
> ◉ Limit your intake of beef, pork, lamb and organ meats. Eat lean fish and poultry.

No comment (but with respect): the late senator Hubert Humphrey's favourite sandwich was reputed to be made with peanut butter, Bologna sausage, cheddar cheese, lettuce and mayonnaise on toasted bread. And all that with a side of ketchup.

Salt

Manufacturers are legally obliged to list salt on the labels of all processed foods, if they add it at all. The catch is that they don't have to tell you *how much* salt they're sprinkling in. Tricky business.

It sure fooled me for a while. I thought I was being good by not salting whatever was canned or packaged. Little did I know that whenever I ate a processed food, I was also downing a lot more salt that I intended to. Let me tell you about salt . . . and hidden salt.

The recommended daily allowance of sodium is only 1100–3300 mg a day for adults. A better top figure, according to the American Health Foundation, is no more than 2000 mg (2 grams). Two grams equals a little under a teaspoon. Most Americans use about 2–4 teaspoons a day.

Salt, chemically speaking, is sodium chloride. About 40 per cent of salt is made up of sodium. It's the sodium part that concerns you, since a high intake of it has been associated with hypertension, kidney problems and stroke.

Even if you don't add salt to processed foods you buy, you're probably getting more sodium than you expected in the package. Here's the bad news.

Campbell's tomato soup, per ½-pint/300-ml serving, has a whopping 1050 mg sodium. Grabbing a fast lunch? One hot dog or a bun with one teaspoon of yellow mustard and about 2 tablespoons of sauerkraut add up to 1160 mg sodium.

Eating instant oatmeal at breakfast gives you about 200 times the sodium of standard rolled oats. Some breakfast cereals have nearly 2½ times the sodium per 1 oz/25 g of Planters Cocktail Peanuts.

The salt shakers are going strong at the canned vegetable factories, too. Del Monte Whole Green Beans, for one, comes in at 925 mg per 7 oz/250 g.

If this gives you indigestion, don't reach for the Eno's or you add another 717 mg sodium per dose. Alka-Seltzer adds 521 mg and Andrews 1000 mg sodium per dose. While laxatives and some sleep aids may solve some of your problems, they're not sodium free.

And watch out for your water. Yes, plain old drinking water. (Not soda water. You *know* that has sodium.) Some cities have water supplies that are high in sodium due to a 'softening process' for hard water. For example, when magnesium and calcium are removed, sodium is substituted.

By the way: if you think soy sauce is a smart alternative to using salt, you should know that 2 teaspoons of soy sauce is equal to a half teaspoon of salt.

What about salt substitutes? Though potassium chloride is the main ingredient in these substitutes, other chemicals are present, too. These are used for a variety of reasons – among them, to decrease bitterness and perk up the flavour.

Salt substitutes pose no problem to healthy folks, but the US Federal Drug Administration and health experts suggest that if you're on a sodium-regulated diet, be sure your doctor okays any salt substitutes. Potassium (or ammonium) salts can be harmful to people who suffer from certain heart disorders and from kidney problems.

Now, as a sodium-conscious consumer, how do you keep away from the stuff? The words 'salt free' on a label aren't enough. If you find the words 'sodium' (along with other compounds, such as sodium saccharine or sodium citrate) or 'brine', the product may be salt free, but it's not sodium free at all.

Some products are obviously salted. Garlic salt, celery salt,

salt pork and onion salt are self-explanatory. You'll also find sodium in baking powder, bicarbonate of soda and self-raising flour. Foods that are pickled or smoked are loaded with sodium, as is any food that contains MSG (monosodium glutamate), a 'flavour enhancer'.

Remember: the more salt you consume, the more water you retain. As little as three-quarters of a teaspoon of salt can add a pound of weight.

Helpful Hints
- Start decreasing your intake of salt by using spices, herbs and lemon in its place. Your taste buds can be retrained to like a lot less salt.
- Check with your local water supply authority to learn the sodium level in your water. If it's high, invest in a sodium filter for the tap. You cook with that water and make tea and coffee.
- Buy low-sodium baking powder and bicarbonate of soda.
- Cut down on processed and canned food and take the time to cook with fresh vegetables.
- Always read the labels on packaged and canned goods. If a product is made with a sodium compound, don't buy it or limit your intake of it.
- Try an interesting tasting salt substitute or kelp powder. Before you use a substitute, such as Selora or Ruthmol, check with your doctor.

No comment: Babe Ruth, the legendary Yankee baseball player, once downed twenty hot dogs before a game.

Caffeine
In 1732, Johann Sebastian Bach paid tribute to the mighty bean by composing 'The Coffee Cantata'. The French statesman Talleyrand, a coffee lover, suggested these qualities for a perfect cup of coffee: 'Black as the devil/Hot as hell/Pure as an angel/Sweet as love.'

Never mind the poetry and music. Coffee's blessed with

a zero calorie count but cursed with caffeine. It's also without nutritional value, interferes with the absorption of B vitamins, and doesn't do much for your system. Caffeine is a stimulant and speeds up fat metabolism, but on the other hand, it can cause mood changes, rapid breathing, rapid heartbeat and palpitations, headaches, tremors, and disturbed sleeping patterns. (And you thought you were just in love!) That's not all. Caffeine also causes kidneys to produce more fluid and your stomach to secrete more acid. Researchers are investigating the effects of a substance in coffee on the development of benign breast lumps (fibrocystic disease) and birth defects.

Most teas aren't as chockful of caffeine as coffee is, but some varieties certainly are. Seems I won't do better with colas, either. Even the one-calorie-per-can colas are high in caffeine count. A 12-oz/350-ml can of Coca-Cola or Pepsi-Cola has between one-third and one-half the caffeine of a cup of coffee. (Plus about eight teaspoons of sugar per can in the non-sugar-free varieties!) There are no decaffeinated colas on the English market.

If I get a headache thinking about this, I'd better examine carefully what I take for it. Many pills, such as Anadin, contain caffeine.

If you or your kids are lovers of another bean – the cocoa bean – you can be getting more caffeine than you want in cocoa, milk chocolate and baking chocolate. Though chocolate has about one-fifth to one-third the amount of caffeine as coffee, it's got a larger dose of another stimulant, theobromine. And chocolate is fattening to boot.

A reasonable dose of caffeine is about 125 mg a day, or what you'd get in one cup of coffee. At that rate some coffee lovers take in 500 mg a day and more.

The amount of caffeine in coffee, tea, colas and chocolate depends on the kind of bean used plus the method of processing, and preparation. How much caffeine are you drinking? *Food Values of Portions Commonly Used*, by Jean A. Pennington and Helen Nichols Church (Harper & Row), cited these figures of caffeine content per ¼-pint/150-ml cup:

> Drip ground coffee: 146 mg per cup with a 137–153 mg
> cup range
> Percolated: 110 mg per cup with a 97–125 mg range
> Instant decaffeinated: 3 mg per cup
> Lipton tea (bagged): 54 mg per cup
> White Rose: 55 mg per cup
> Coca-Cola: 65 mg per 12-oz/350-ml can
> Pepsi-Cola: 36 mg per 12-oz/350-ml can
> Carnation instant cocoa mix: 13 mg per package

Helpful Hints

- Keep coffee consumption down to one cup a day; same for tea.
- Switch to decaffeinated coffees and teas. If you can find them, buy coffees that have been decaffeinated with a water process instead of the chemically treated ones.
- Even better, switch to coffee and tea substitutes. Most grain beverages, such as Instant Postum, have about 12 calories per cup and contain some nutritional value.
- Drink, if you must, sweet soft drinks that are caffeine free. Even better, sip salt-free seltzers or soda water with a twist of lime. You get no overload from sugar or caffeine from these.
- If you're tempted to eat chocolate, remember that not only aren't the fats and calories good for you – neither is the caffeine.

Sugar

A few hundred years ago, sugar was sold in pharmacies. If you got some, it was because sugar was considered more a medicine than a treat. For some of us sugar-holics, it *is* a drug.

It's also delicious. But as TV's 'Rhoda' once said about chocolate: 'I don't know why I'm eating this. I might as well apply it directly to my hips.' A teaspoon of sugar isn't fattening. But for those of us who consume up to 500 calories or more a day from one sort of sugar or another, it's dangerous.

White sugar isn't the only sweetener we down by the bucketful. There's golden syrup, treacle, molasses, maple sugar, honey, fructose, maltose, lactose, and light and dark brown sugars and icing sugar. It appears to be everywhere, whether you want it or not.

You know if you eat a toffee, you're eating sugar. But to suit the nation's sweet tooth (cavity-prone), manufacturers add it to hot dogs, breakfast cereals, some processed foods, salad dressings, chewing gums, ketchups, even coatings for food such as crumbs.

Sugar, like starch, is a carbohydrate and a source of energy. A gram of carbohydrate amounts to 4 calories – the same as protein. Simple sugar (as in a chocolate bar) is the quickest source of energy, but it's not long lasting. You get a rapid peak boost when glucose is transported to your cells by insulin, but often your pancreas secretes an excess of insulin and releases more than you need. Your blood sugar drops and you feel worse. To feel better, you eat more sweets. And the cycle starts again. It's much smarter to eat complex carbohydrates (like pasta or bread) which take longer to get into your bloodstream.

The total amount of calories you eat, not the proportion of calories made up of sugar, is what makes you gain weight. The problem is that sugar addicts can eat a *lot* of sweets – amd therefore a *lot* of calories.

If you want to lose weight, sugar's gotta go.

Helpful Hints
- You'd have to eat eight or nine apples (about 3 lb/1.5 kg) to get the same calories as 5 oz/150 g of milk chocolate. One apple is more satisfying for bulk and sweetness. *Eat fruit!*
- Read the package labels on all foods you buy and check for corn sweeteners, lactose, dextrose, sucrose, fructose,

honey or molasses on the labels. If any sweetener is listed as one of the first three ingredients, the product has a high sugar content.

- Do not keep a sugar bowl on the table. Develop a taste for foods without sugar.
- Increase your use of tangy spices like cinnamon, ginger, cardamom, and nutmeg.
- Don't bake rich desserts or buy any sweets – even if they're on sale. If it's not in the house, you can't nibble.
- Cut down on soft drinks with sugar (they have up to eight teaspoons of sugar per 12-oz/350-ml can).
- Dried fruits sound promising but they're loaded with sugar. Five dried apricots have the equivalent of about 4 teaspoons of sugar. 1½ oz/40 g raisins have about 4 teaspoons worth of sugar.

Food for thought: the American Dream: getting rich. The American Nightmare: getting fat.

Alcohol

The only occasion I know of that doesn't 'call for a drink' is breakfast. Brunch is close, but no cigar.

Drinking is supposed to make you feel happy, relaxed, a little looser with your words and deeds, social and lots of fun. As we all know, too much booze, and you're on 'tilt'. There's no fun in that.

Alcohol is an amazing liquid. It's on your food exchange list as a fat, but it's actually in it's own category, since its a drug *and* a carbohydrate. (Alcoholic beverages are fermented from fruits and grains.) When it's metabolized, you get twice the calories per gram as from starch or sugar. It also works on you faster than the proverbial speeding bullet. Ethanol is what makes it happen. Ethanol is an ingredient in alcohol that shoots through your system via your bloodstream. Your liver works like mad to break ethanol down and defuse it, but it can only process so much an hour.

What happens then? Ethanol starts to collect in body

tissues. When it hits your brain, you begin to feel light-headed. Give your body a small glassful of vodka (brandy, Scotch) and you're feeling good. A little more and you may trip over the sofa. After five drinks, you're officially intoxicated.

Too much alcohol over an extended period of time can wreck your body. It can accelerate ageing (who needs that?), make you forgetful, and cause wide mood swings, to name a few results. You can develop skin sensitivity so great that even a light touch hurts. It can cause problems with blood clotting and high blood pressure.

Alcohol is also very caloric, which is why I'm talking about it here.

One fluid ounce usually equals a shot. The home barman may use a jigger, which is 1½ ounces. Think about it. When's the last time anyone served a one-shot drink? Most of them end up being two-shot drinks. Double the calories.

The caloric content of distilled liquors depends on the percentage of alcohol. The proof is twice the alcohol percentage. (80 proof = 40 per cent alcohol.) The following values apply to all brands of Scotch, rye, brandy, rum, gin, tequila and vodka.

80 proof 1 fl oz/25 ml: 70 calories	1½ fl oz/40 ml: 105 calories
86 proof 1 fl oz/25 ml: 75 calories	1½ fl oz/40 ml: 112 calories
90 proof 1 fl oz/25 ml: 79 calories	1½ fl oz/40 ml: 118 calories
94 proof 1 fl oz/25 ml: 83 calories	1½ fl oz/40 ml: 124 calories
100 proof 1 fl oz/25 ml: 89 calories	1½ fl oz/40 ml: 133 calories

Let's see what we've got in one glass here (refilled twice). Three Scotch and waters (80 proof, double shots) add up to 420 empty calories. And if you prefer sweet drinks, you're in big trouble. Don't even bring that glass to your lips. Piña coladas, for example, should be outlawed: 6 fl oz/175 ml total 480 calories.

Drinking in moderation is certainly okay. In fact, a 1974 government report said that moderate drinkers are more likely to live longer and have fewer heart attacks than people who don't drink at all, who've stopped drinking, or drink way too much. As far as I know, this report hasn't been challenged.

Helpful Hints

- Don't let two or three drinks (beer, wine or the tougher spirits) substitute for food.
- Carbonated wines like champagne or drinks mixed with soda get you higher faster. Those bubbles do it. Straight alcohol is fast, but the carbonation in your stomach makes you absorb the alcohol into your blood faster.
- If you're feeling low, a drink will affect you quicker than if you're feeling okay.
- One drink won't hurt. Choose a lower calorie drink (like 'light' beer or white wine or the lower calorie wines) and nurse it.

In case you wondered: there's a trace amount of alcohol in bread.

Diet Pills

When you have a fat problem, what sounds better than a pill that will take it all away? Take two or twenty, and the fat flies off. The truth is that diet pills are about as critical to *long-term* weight loss as the wrist corsage – and a lot more dangerous. The pounds may go, but your health may well depart along with them.

Diet pills used to be available by prescription only. They were called 'uppers', or technically, amphetamines. The main reason amphetamines worked was because they suppressed the appetite centre in the brain. You just didn't feel like eating. A few problems resulted – psychological dependence, mental disturbances and elevation of blood pressure. Maybe you weren't eating or overeating, but you didn't feel like living either.

We have progress to thank for a new diet pill being tested that doesn't work with amphetamines, but a chemical that's just as bad. If you're a crossword puzzle fan, you might like to know it's called phenylpropanolomine. This chemical has been approved by American authorities because it's supposedly not habit-forming and it's less likely for a person to become psychologically dependent on it. But a lot of people believe in diet pills. Dieting Americans bought about $200 million worth of the stuff in 1980.

Phenylpropanolomine works like amphetamines. It's a stimulant and constricts blood vessels. Your body takes it as an appetite suppressant. There have been various studies on this 'wonder' pill. Pill-takers have reported restlessness, irritability, elevation of blood pressure, sleep problems, mental disturbances, and in some cases, seizures and strokes.

There's another reason not to take these pills: some brands contain caffeine, too – as much in one pill as two cups of coffee. If your heart isn't pounding from the phenyl-propanolomine, the caffeine may set it off.

Here's the point: diet pills do not work for long-term weight loss. The brain adapts to the drug and, being smart, soon ignores its messages. The only answer for long-term weight loss is a conscious effort to change your eating habits and attitudes about food and . . . I guess you have my message by now: *exercise*.

Helpful Hints

- Even if you don't feel any of the adverse effects of these pills when you take them, and if you lose some weight because of them, will you be able to keep the weight off? If you're a 'yo-yo' weight gainer, the answer's no.
- Don't buy these pills. Don't even read the backs of the packages. They may tempt you.

What would we do without Art: on describing a 'powder mix' diet for the *New York Herald Tribune* some years back, Art Buchwald commented, 'The powder is mixed with water and tastes exactly like powder mixed with water.'

Restaurant Food

Bear with me a minute on this. George Washington once said that the state of New Jersey was a 'nest of infamous turncoats'. Don't ask me who told me this or why I remembered it, but it sure fits what I'm going to tell you about salad bars. There among the greenery (not in Jersey, but at the salad bar) are stainless steel containers on ice filled with 'infamous turncoats' – grated, diced, julienned, pickled, fried, and creamed foods. Think of some of them as traitors, not your pals, and you'll win the war on fat.

I'm not against the idea of salad bars, just what salad bars are shovelling out. What happens to some of us is this: we equate salad bars with 'as much as you want'. Salad bar owners know they have a good thing going: their places draw customers. Customers think they have a better thing going because they can pile their plates sky-high.

But do you want to?

Let's take a walk down salad bar lane. You'll usually find:

chopped eggs	green peppers	pickled beetroot
raw spinach	lettuce	grated carrots
sliced onions	spring onions	bean sprouts
hard cheese chunks	grated cheddar	creamed herring
bacon shreds	croutons	anchovies
sliced tomatoes	pickled mushrooms	olives
chickpeas	Parmesan cheese	diced raw courgette
pickled herring		

All this is followed by at least 6 vats of salad dressing and 6 ladles of mayonnaise.

One half of this list is good for you; the other half sends

your low-cal lunch into the 'steak and brew' category not only in terms of calories, but also fat or sodium intake.

Heres the plan; skip the pickled foods, creamed herring, and bacon. They're either high in fat, salt or both. Skip the chunked and grated cheeses and eggs. Pass up the chickpeas and croutons and pretend 'olive' is only a colour. Absolutely do not dip into the Roquefort, French, Russian, Green Goddess, Thousand Island, or any other loving-hands-in-the-kitchen homemade creamy dressings.

So, you say, what's left that's good? For one, your ability to toss a salad that will be filling and still be around 100 calories or so. Your salad will consist of greens, onions, grated carrots, four slices of tomato, green pepper and a mere sprinkling of grated Parmesan cheese.

Helpful Hints

- Don't drop in a 'taste' of bacon or creamed herring. Cheating is cheating, even if it's by a half teaspoon.
- Mix your own dressing with their lemon wedges and some spices. Ask if they have any low-calorie dressings. Better yet, bring your own packets along.

The Continentals

As far as I know George Washington never said anything interesting about French food, but if he tasted it, he probably thought it was pretty *bon*. Who wouldn't? It's a knockout, if you have no weight problem. French food is loaded with cream sauces, butter and wine; the desserts are to die from, but are they rich!

Italian, Spanish and German restaurants are not without potential for the danger list – their dishes, too, are made with loads of oil, cheese, and fatty or overly sweet ingredients. Though I'll be dealing with the unromantic side to the French restaurant, follow the same guidelines in Helpful Hints, below, for any restaurant.

Some dishes appear low-cal but are actually killers in calories. Salmon mousse is one. It's made with eggs and cream. Avoid any 'au gratin' dishes – that means it's got baked cheese on top. 'Cordon bleu' sounds classy, but that means the dish is stuffed with ham and cheese. 'Provençal' means it's made with garlic (that's okay) and olive oil or butter (not so okay). 'Terrines' will really get you. They're just pâté in another form, made with minced duck and pork plus other high-calorie ingredients. 'Pommes frites' are only french fries.

No sauce in a French restaurant is a good sauce – and I'm not talking about the quality of the cookery. Whether it's 'béchamel', 'béarnaise', or 'hollandaise', pass it by. 'Vinaigrette' dressing is vinegar and olive oil with seasonings.

Now that you're ready to despair over never entering a French restaurant again, don't. You can. Look for these key words when you order a dish: 'grillade', grilled; 'rôti', roasted; 'au jus', in its own juice; 'au naturel', without any additions, sauces or tampering with; and 'crudités', raw, julienned vegetables without dressing.

Helpful Hints

- When a menu is in another language, ask exactly what each dish is, what's in it, and how it was prepared. If your waiter lifts an eyebrow at you, lift one back. Insist on knowing what you're ordering and don't let a guy in a dinner jacket push you around.
- Request that fish be grilled with no butter.
- Ask that sauces remain in the kitchen, not be spooned liberally on to your plate.
- If dinner comes with fried or heavily buttered oven-fried potatoes, ask for a vegetable side dish (like asparagus) or tiny boiled potatoes. If the waiter insists there are no substitutions, insist there are. If Princess Di showed up, they'd find some for her.
- Skip any rich desserts and order strawberries or melon in season.

Coffee Shops

Coffee shops are conveniently located, whip up the kind of food you know and love, and the prices are reasonable. However, there's something about coffee shops that immediately makes me think 'fat'. Maybe it has to do with that open grill so many have. Everything's cooked on it: toasted sandwiches, burgers, pancakes, eggs, bacon and sausages. With plenty of grease.

Sandwiches are usually a big item here: tuna with mayonnaise; chicken or egg salad; bacon, lettuce, and tomato on white toast. French frying onion rings ruins onions, a perfectly good low-cal vegetable. The cakes are usually about 9 inches high and look as if they're made from sawdust and food colouring. The pies, as my friend Roger says, are either strawberry, apple or cherry 'effect'. They're so loaded with flour and sugar, you just get the 'effect' of eating real fruit pie.

The also offer a 'dieter's plate': a scoop of cottage cheese with half a canned cling peach, a burger without the bun, a scoop of coleslaw dripping with mayonnaise, and a carrot curl. Okay on the carrot curl and cottage cheese. You don't need all that protein nor the sugar in the canned peach. You'd actually be better off eating the bun, which you really want and is a source of complex carbohydrates, an appropriate balance for the meal.

There's something friendly about the coffee shop. You want to order friendly foods like salami on rye. But coffee shops are about as concerned with low-cal dining as the French restaurant. It's up to you to say no.

Helpful Hints

- Order sliced chicken, turkey or roast beef without bread or dressings. Trim the fat from the beef.
- Order tuna in brine on a bed of lettuce with a side order of tomatoes, sliced.
- Order a baked potato instead of french or home fries.

- Skip the puddings or hi-cal desserts. Order half a grapefruit or melon balls.
- Ask them to grill the burgers or grill an open-faced cheese and tomato sandwich instead of frying them on the grill.
- Ask for melba toast instead of bread.
- Ask for sandwiches with lettuce and tomato. These make the sandwich thicker without adding many calories.
- Don't sit around and dawdle. You may be tempted to order a goodie.

Organic, Health, and Natural Foods

I forget the newspaper I once saw this story in, but I like the point it makes. A traditionally minded mother wanted to buy her hip, vegetarian daughter a string of pearls. 'Gross,' said the daughter, or words to that effect. 'Why?' said the mother. 'They're organic.'

Pearls are organic, vegetables are organic, even mother and daughter are organic. The question is: are 'organic' foods better for you than the commercial 'non-organic' foods sold at the supermarket? Some say yes; others, like me, say no. Good food is good food. If you're smart enough to serve the frozen spinach and throw out the plastic boiling bag, you know the difference between organic and non-organic.

What's all the flap about organic or 'health' foods? So far, there's no legal definition of health foods or of the term 'organic'. Organic is supposed to describe food that's been grown without pesticides, growth hormones, or chemically based fertilizers when the crop was on the vine. Personally, I'm not mad about eating foods that are coated with pesticides, but the truth is that I don't, and you don't. As it turns out, the Government has regulations and guidelines about pesticide residues on foods. The amount of these residues is usually infinitesimal.

It is true that most processed foods lose many of their nutrients, and that some foods retain traces of pesticides and are packed with preservatives and additives. But, so far, no one's found any evidence that health foods or organic foods are better for you or any safer.

Organically grown crops are not necessarily more nutritious. A peach grown in California by a commercial producer using chemical fertilizers is as nutritious (more, in some cases) as one grown with manure or compost. What makes fruits or vegetables nutritious is the genetic nature, the climate, the nutrients available for growth, and the stage of maturity at which they are harvested.

There have been lots of tests that show that organic foods have little (and often no) difference in taste, appearance, and nutritional value from the commercial product. The biggest difference is – you guessed it – the price.

You may be paying two to three times as much for organically grown fruits and vegetables as what you pay at your local produce counter. Why the cost? Organic farming takes more labour, so for those honest farmers who make a living this way, I can understand the higher prices. The second reason is not so homespun. Because of the trend towards buying organically grown foods, some crooks around are jacking up the price of commercially grown stuff by calling it 'organic'.

Here's another scoop on health foods. They're often loaded with fat, sugar, salt and cholesterol. Take the ever-popular muesli – it can be one of the highest calorie breakfast cereals you eat. It's got about four times the calories as, say, ordinary corn flakes, thanks to its dried fruit and honey. Some carob (chocolate substitute) bars are made with palm oil – another highly saturated fat. A health food fruit and nut dessert bar has 344 calories per 4 oz/100 g, as many as most similar commercial ones. (Don't buy any of them.)

If you're on a diet, you may not buy health foods, but what about 'natural' foods? Personally, I have no reason to doubt that my Unsweetened Grapefruit Juice is natural. (It sure wasn't concocted in a lab.) My skim milk Jarlsberg cheese is natural. So is Quaker Oats. How come the companies are hawking 'natural' as if real food with real ingredients were just invented? Because it *sounds* so good.

Okay. You buy a food that says 'natural' on the label. Sometimes it is. Other times, you read the label and your jaw drops. Right there in black and white, they admit it contains any or all of the following: additives, sugar, salt, MSG (monosodium glutamate), vegetable gums, partially hydrogenated oils, bleached white flour or food colouring.

Some of the manufacturers say that sugar, white flour, food colouring, and all the other stuff they're dropping in is 'natural' or natural enough. (That reminds me of my friend Marilyn, the 'natural' beauty, with her nose reduction, chin enhancement, capped teeth and frosted hair.)

As with organic and health foods, there's no legal definition of natural yet. Generally, it's understood as food that's free of preservatives, additives and artificial flavours. 'Natural' may just mean that the guy at the cheese factory is using real cheese in a product instead of processed; it doesn't have to mean he isn't using some sort of preservative in the prepacking.

You can have 100 per cent natural foods, but many items would rot or go rancid without some preservatives. It's not the best news to know your food has preservatives in it, but then again, you're assured of buying food that's edible and safe.

Helpful Hints

- Watch out for 'natural' enzymes, 'miracle' weeds, or extracts of herbs, beans or plants that promise weight loss or offer themselves up as food substitutes.
- Beware those tempting bins of carob-coated raisins and nuts, honeyed dried bananas, coconut chips and dried fruits. They look tempting, but are high in calories.
- Watch out for 'nut' substitutes. They're made with saturated oils.
- Don't buy protein powders, cake or pancake mixes, 'protein cookies', or any other product without checking

the label to see the fat content (and type of fat), sugar, salt, and other ingredient levels. You may just be getting higher calories at higher cost.

- A slightly shrivelled-looking apple at a health food store isn't necessarily a better apple. You're probably better off buying from a reputable produce dealer. Just wash the apple off before eating.
- Read all labels of foods calling themselves natural.

Cigarettes
I know, this is a diet book. Why am I mentioning cigarettes? Because they're killers, like fat. I know it, but I still smoke. I figure if I could finally lose weight after a long battle, I can stop smoking. That's my next project.

Got any ideas?

19. Formerly Fattening Recipes

One way to reduce the calorie count in what you're eating is to add air or water to the food, increasing bulk without increasing food value. Another is by simply cutting down on your portions. In recipes, you can generally reduce the calorie count by decreasing either the fat or sugar content. I use one or more of these principles to adapt recipes for entertaining. I like having company, and I don't think dieting has to turn you into a hermit. It doesn't have to mean dietetic disaster for you or your guests. Look over these recipes for use as is or for ideas to cut calories in some of your favourite dishes.

BRIDAL SHOWER
Pink Grapefruit Punch
Pastel Dessert
or
Strawberry Glazed Cheesecake

Pink Grapefruit Punch
8 8-oz/225-g servings (42 calories each)

1 10-oz/275-g package unsweetened frozen strawberries
1 litre/36 fl oz slimline American ginger ale
1¼ pints/750 ml unsweetened grapefruit juice
mint leaves (optional)

Purée juice and strawberries in blender until smooth. Add ginger ale and stir gently. Garnish with fresh mint leaves.

- Sugar calories are saved by using low-sugar juice, low-cal ginger ale and unsweetened strawberries.

Pastel Dessert
8 squares (140 calories each)

3 oz/75 g digestive biscuit crumbs
1 T. margarine or butter
8 fl oz/225 ml evaporated skim milk, boiled 20 minutes
  in unopened can and cooled
¾ pint/425 ml ice cream sorbet

Melt margarine or butter and mix with biscuit crumbs, reserving 1½ T. crumbs for topping. Turn into 8 inch/20 cm square cake tin. Cool crust in freezer. Chill skim milk, bowl, and beaters until almost frozen, then whip. Quickly fold in softened sorbet and spread over crumbs. Sprinkle reserved crumbs over top and freeze until firm.

- Thin crust, with reduced fat and no sugar, saves calories.
- Whipping evaporated skim milk (200 calories per cup, unwhipped) saves 220 calories compared to whipped cream (421 calories per cup).

Strawberry Glazed Cheesecake
8 slices (140 calories each)

2 T. margarine
3 oz/75 g digestive biscuit crumbs
2 fl oz/60 ml water
½ tsp. grated orange rind
8 oz/225 g low-fat cottage cheese
⅛ pint/75 ml evaporated skim milk
2 envelopes (2 T.) unflavoured gelatine
3 T. orange juice concentrate
2 egg whites
⅛ tsp. salt

2 T. sugar
8 oz/225 g fresh unsweetened frozen strawberries, mashed

Preheat oven to 400° F/200° C, gas mark 6. Melt margarine in 9 inch/22.5 cm springform cake tin. Mix in crumbs and press over bottom of pan. Bake 5 to 7 minutes and set aside to cool. In a blender, purée cottage cheese with milk until smooth and chill. In a saucepan over low heat, mix 2 T. orange juice concentrate, 2 T. water, 1 T. sugar, orange rind, and 1½ envelopes (1 T. plus 1½ tsp.) gelatine, stirring constantly until gelatine is dissolved. Remove from heat and let stand at room temperature. In a medium bowl, beat egg whites with salt until stiff. Fold in gelatine mixture and cottage cheese mixture. Pour over crumb crust and refrigerate. When set, add strawberry glaze.

Glaze
In a saucepan over low heat, mix ½ envelope (1½ tsp.) gelatine, 2 T. water, 1 T. sugar and 1 T. orange juice concentrate until gelatine is dissolved. Remove from heat, stir in mashed strawberries. Spread mixture evenly over cheesecake and refrigerate until firm.

- Fat content is decreased by substituting skim milk and low-fat cottage cheese.
- Sugar kept to minimum in crust, cake and glaze.
- Portions are slightly smaller than traditional cheesecake, which is 320 calories per slice.

FOOTBALL BUFFET
Raw Vegetables
Assorted Dips
Hot Tomato Bouillon
Lasagna
French Bread with Chive Butter *or* Margarine
Green Salad
with Special Vinaigrette Dressing and
Herbed Croutons
Cream Puffs

Blue Cheese Dip
16 1-oz/25-ml servings (20 calories per serving)

6 oz/175 g low-fat cottage cheese
4 oz/100 g blue cheese, crumbled
6 fl oz/175 ml plain yogurt
1 T. chopped parsley

Purée cottage cheese and yogurt in blender until smooth. Mix in remaining ingredients. Chill.

Cheddar Dip
16 1-oz/25-ml servings (24 calories per serving)

2 oz/50 g grated cheddar cheese
6 oz/175 g plain low-fat yogurt
¼ tsp. dry mustard
2 tsp. chives, minced
¼ tsp. paprika

Combine all ingredients. Chill.

Hot and Spicy Dip
24 1-oz/25-ml servings (10 calories per serving)

8 oz/225 g plain low-fat yogurt
⅛ pint/75 ml barbecue sauce
2 tsp. grated, bottled horseradish (not cream)
1 tsp. finely chopped chives or onion
2 tsp. prepared mustard
⅛ tsp. Worcestershire sauce
2 T. finely chopped celery

Combine all ingredients. Chill.

- Low-fat cottage cheese (200 calories per 8 oz/225 g) and yogurt (140 calories per 8 oz/225 g) are substituted for soured cream (420 calories per 8 fl oz/225 ml).
- Fresh vegetables can include tomato wedges, celery, spring onions, mushrooms, carrots, green pepper. Have you tried courgette, cauliflower, broccoli, turnips, beetroot, and Chinese leaves raw? You're avoiding the high fat and salt content of crackers when you serve vegetables in their place.

Hot Tomato Bouillon
8 8-oz/225-ml servings (35 calories per serving)

8 beef stock cubes
3¼ pints/1.8 litres tomato juice

Pour 1½ pints/900 ml hot water into a large saucepan with stock cubes; heat until melted. Then add tomato juice and keep on flame until warm.

- This substitutes for high-calorie mixed drinks and gets you just as warm.

French Bread with Chive Butter or Margarine
64 calories per ½ inch/1 cm slice

Use ½ tsp. butter per slice, adding 1 tsp. finely chopped chives to each 4 tsp. butter. Wrap the whole loaf in foil and warm in the oven after you have removed the lasagna and are letting it set.

● Pre-buttering the bread controls the size of the portion.

Special Vinaigrette Dressing
16 1-T. servings (30 calories each)

3 T. vegetable oil
5 T. wine or herb vinegar
2 T. lemon juice
5 T. water
1½ tsp. Dijon-style mustard
1 garlic clove, crushed
1 tsp. crushed tarragon
1 T. finely chopped shallots or chives
¼ tsp. paprika
⅛ tsp. ground pepper
salt to taste (optional)

Mix well in a tightly covered jar. Store in the refrigerator.

● Oil in this dressing is kept to a minimum, and in its place are low-calorie extenders such as vinegar, lemon juice, and water.

Lasagna
8 servings (350 calories per serving)

¾ lb/340 g extra-lean minced beef
2 garlic cloves, crushed
28 fl oz/850 ml thick tomato juice (simmer down 1¾ pints/1 litre juice)
1 6-oz/175-g can tomato paste
½ tsp. fennel seeds
1 bay leaf
1 T. parsley, chopped
16 oz/454 g low-fat cottage cheese
8 oz/225 g mozzarella cheese, grated or crumbled
1 egg, beaten
8 oz/225 g lasagna rectangles (about 12)
1½ tsp. oregano
ground black pepper to taste

Preheat oven to 375° F/190° C, gas mark 5.

In a large frying pan, brown mince with garlic and drain off any fat. Add tomato juice, tomato paste, and all seasonings except parsley. Prepare lasagna according to package directions, drain, and rinse with cold water in a colander. With electric beater, whip cottage cheese with egg and parsley. Cover the bottom of a 9×13 inch/225×325 mm baking tin with half the meat sauce. Cover with half the lasagna, overlapping to fit. Layer with half the cottage cheese mixture, then half the remaining meat sauce and half the grated mozzarella cheese. Repeat the layers. Bake for 40–45 minutes. Remove from oven and let stand for 10 minutes to set.

- This has half the calories of traditional homemade lasagna because we have used no oil, a small quantity of lean meat, low-fat cheese, and a small quantity of tomato paste.
- Fennel seeds help sharpen the taste without the calories of sausage.

Cream Puffs
8 servings (150 calories each)

2 oz/50 g butter or margarine
4 fl oz/120 ml boiling water
2 oz/50 g flour
¼ tsp. nutmeg
2 whole eggs

Filling
4 tsp. cornflour
2 T. sugar
8 fl oz/225 ml skim milk
1 egg yolk
½ tsp. vanilla

Preheat oven to 350° F/180° C, gas mark 4.

In a medium saucepan, heat butter or margarine with water until melted. Add flour and nutmeg and beat until mixture is smooth and pulls away from sides of pan cleanly. Remove from heat and add eggs, one at a time, until dough forms a thick, shiny paste. Drop rounded tablespoonful 2 inches/5 cm apart on a baking sheet covered with Bakewell paper. (You should have enough batter for eight puffs.) Bake for 40 minutes or until puffs are lightly browned, then cool on rack.

Filling
Combine cornflour and sugar in a medium-sized saucepan. Add milk over heat, stirring constantly, until mixture thickens and bubbles. Beat egg yolk slightly in a small bowl, then stir it into the cornflour mixture until smooth. Heat two minutes longer, stirring constantly. Remove from heat and add vanilla. Cool.

Preparation

Split cooled puffs and fill with vanilla filling. Optional: top cream puffs with a few sliced strawberries or blackberries, or a slice of peach, pineapple, or banana.

- We cut the calories per puff from the usual 250 calories to 150 calories by reducing the sugar and using low-fat milk.

HOLIDAY BARBECUE
Shish Kebabs
Fruit Salad
French Bread with Herb Butter *or* Margarine
Angel Food Cake with Fruited Whipped Topping

Shish Kebabs
8 servings (300 calories per serving)

1½ lb/775 g lean roast beef, cubed (3 oz/75 g per diet serving)*
4 green peppers, sliced
8 tomatoes, chopped
24 small white onions
4 courgettes (1-1½ inch/2-3 cm in diameter) cut in ¾-inch/2-cm slices

Marinade
¾ pint/425 ml red wine
2 T. soy sauce
2 T. Dijon mustard
4 fl oz/120 ml lemon juice
4 T. cornflour

Mix marinade ingredients and pour over meat cubes. Refrigerate several hours or overnight. To assemble on 8 skewers, alternate meat and vegetables (allowing about ½

* You may want to increase the amount of beef for non-dieters.

green pepper, 1 tomato, 3 onions and a half a courgette per portion). Grill on barbecue or in oven approximately 15 minutes, turning once or twice. Baste with remaining marinade during cooking.

- There's very little oil in this marinade, and we've used a very lean cut of meat to save fat calories. Substitute chicken for beef and you save another 100 calories per serving.
- The vegetables accompanying the meat are also low calorie.

Fruit Salad
8 servings (75 calories per serving)

8 oz/225 g pineapple chunks (fresh or packed in natural juice and drained)
3 oz/75 g fresh green grapes
2 nectarines, sliced
8 oz/225 g melon balls (honeydew, cantaloupe, watermelon, or mixture)
1 banana, sliced
3 oz/75 g orange juice concentrate, melted
¼ tsp. ground ginger

Toss fruit in a bowl together with a mixture of ginger and orange juice concentrate. Refrigerate and serve.

- Using fresh, unsweetened fruits and orange juice concentrate instead of a honey dressing or heavy sugar syrup saves about 50 calories per serving.

Angel Food Cake with Fruited Whipped Topping
8 slices (140 calories per serving)

1 packet Angel food cake mix
6 fl oz/175 ml evaporated skim milk, whipped
1 lb/450 g fresh or frozen strawberries or raspberries, sliced
grated lemon rind (optional)

Prepare cake according to package and bake in 10 inch/250 mm tube cake tin. Cool. Freeze half of the cake and slice other half into 8 portions. Chill evaporated skim milk, beaters, and bowl until almost frozen, then whip. Fold in fruit and grated lemon rind. Top each slice with ⅛ of mixture.

- Angel food cake contains less fat than most cakes, so it has 50 to 100 less calories per serving.
- You save another 50 calories by substituting the fruited topping for frosting or whipped cream.

DINNER PARTY
Herbed Chicken
Low-Cal Twice-Baked Potatoes
Nutty Green Beans
Minted Fruit Compôte
Popovers
Pumpkin Soufflés

Herbed Chicken
4 servings (280 calories per serving)

2 lb/1.1 kg boneless chicken breasts, skinned
3 oz/75 g chopped spring onions
1 T. vegetable oil
1 T. butter or margarine

1 tsp. dried rosemary
1½ tsp. chopped parsley
⅛ tsp. paprika
3 oz/75 g tuna, drained and rinsed

In a large frying pan, melt butter or margarine with oil and sauté chicken and onion about 3 minutes. Drain any remaining fat. Add remaining ingredients, then lower heat and simmer, covered, for 30 minutes or until chicken is tender.

- By removing the skin, using a minimal amount of fat in this recipe, and eliminating high-calorie gravy, you keep the calories to a minimum.

Twice-Baked Potatoes
4 servings (80 calories per serving)

2 medium baking potatoes, baked
4 oz/100 g plain low-fat yogurt
4 tsp. Parmesan cheese
1 tsp. dried grated onion
paprika

Cut potatoes in half lengthwise and scoop out cooked portion, keeping skin intact. Mash potato, then add yogurt and whip with electric mixer until fluffy. Fold in Parmesan cheese and onion. Place potato skin halves on a flat baking tray or sheet and fill with potato mixture. Sprinkle each with paprika. Bake 20–30 minutes at 350° F/180° C, gas mark 4 or until top is lightly browned and potato is heated through. (Filled potato shells may be made the day before and covered and refrigerated or frozen for later use.)

- These moist potatoes are tasty and 100 calories less than the usual twice-baked potato recipe, thanks to the yogurt/ Parmesan cheese combination being substituted for more

231

fattening ingredients. They also eliminate the need for gravy.

Nutty Green Beans
4 servings (50 calories per serving)

¾ lb/340 g cut green beans
1 T. butter or margarine
1 tsp. lemon juice
¼ tsp. garlic powder
½ oz/15 g flaked almonds

Steam beans until just tender. Toss in serving bowl together with margarine, lemon juice, and garlic powder. Sprinkle almonds on top.

● Garlic and lemon juice help spark the taste of green beans without adding salt, and fat is kept to a minimum.

Minted Fruit Compôte
4 servings (100 calories per serving)

14 oz/400 g fresh pineapple, cubed
2 medium oranges, peeled and diced
4 tsp. frozen orange juice concentrate
4 tsp. water
2–3 drops mint essence
fresh mint leaves (optional)

Mix ingredients and garnish with fresh mint leaves. May be served hot or cold.

● Fresh fruit and unsweetened juice keeps calorie count down.

Popovers
6 popovers (65 calories apiece)

4 fl oz/120 ml skim milk
1 egg, beaten
2 oz/50 g flour
1 T. melted butter or margarine
⅛ tsp. salt

Preheat oven to 450° F/230° C, gas mark 8. Spray a 6-cup deep bun tin with vegetable cooking oil. Beat milk, margarine, salt, and flour together until smooth. Add egg, beating lightly. Divide batter into six cups and bake at once. After 15 minutes lower heat to 350° F/180° C, gas mark 4 (do not open oven), and bake about 20 minutes longer until sides of popovers are firm. Serve at once.

● Low-fat milk cuts some of the calories, and these popovers are meant to be slightly smaller than usual.

Pumpkin Soufflés
4 servings (54 calories per serving)

Topping
2 fl oz/60 ml evaporated skim milk, boiled for 20 minutes in unopened can and cooled
1 tsp. frozen orange juice concentrate

6 oz/175 g canned pumpkin
2 egg whites, slightly beaten
1 T. sugar
8 fl oz/225 ml skim milk
⅛ tsp. ginger
⅛ tsp. cloves
¼ tsp. cinnamon
⅛ tsp. nutmeg

Make topping first: chill evaporated skim milk, bowl and

beater almost to freezing. Whisk milk until almost whipped, then add frozen orange juice concentrate and complete whipping. Chill until ready to serve. Purée pumpkin with egg whites, sugar, milk and spices in a blender and divide into 4 small custard cups. Set custard cups in a large deep frying pan filled with water within ½ inch/1 cm of the top of the custard cups. Heat water just to simmer over moderate heat, cover, and steam for 15 minutes or until soufflés are just set. Refrigerate until well chilled. Divide topping among four custard cups and serve.

SUMMER PICNIC
Pitta Bread with Chicken Salad
Fresh Fruit
Raw Vegetables
Spiced Meringue Drops
Ice Tea with Lemon

Pitta Bread with Chicken Salad
Makes 1 sandwich (150 calories per *half*)

1 5-inch/12.5-cm whole wheat pitta from health food stores
3½ oz/85 g white chicken meat, cooked and diced
1 small stalk of celery, chopped
½ tomato, chopped
2 cos lettuce leaves, chopped
1 radish, chopped
2 tsp. Special Vinaigrette Dressing (see page 225)

Toss filling ingredients and pack in plastic container. Fill at the picnic so bread won't become soggy.

- Skinless chicken is a low-fat, good source of protein.
- Special Vinaigrette is a much lower calorie substitute for the usual mayonnaise used in a salad like this.
- Vegetables add texture and bulk with minimal calories.

Fresh Fruit and Raw Vegetables
● Take advantage of the season by buying a variety of items that are plentiful and cheap. Serving without sauce and dressing cuts your calorie intake substantially.

Spiced Meringue Drops
30 drops (14 calories apiece)

2 egg whites
⅛ tsp. salt
4 oz/100 g sugar
½ tsp. cinnamon
⅛ tsp. nutmeg
¼ tsp. ginger
pinch of ground gloves

Preheat oven to 250° F/120° C, gas mark ¼.

Beat egg whites and salt until they form soft peaks. Gradually beat in sugar and spices. Drop about 1 inch/2.5 cm apart on to non-stick baking sheets. Bake 2 hours or until drops are very light brown and crisp.

● Using only the egg white and not the yolk cuts fat calories dramatically.
● These cookies are quite low in sugar.

20. Alternatives and Substitutes: Or, How to Eat an Egg Without Eating an Egg

I know how it feels to read an article telling you that when you crave a hot fudge sundae, eat half an apple instead. Only a person who's never eaten a hot fudge sundae would be able to say that. There is no appropriate substitute for a hot fudge sundae except maybe a hot caramel sundae. Forget either one while you're dieting. (And remember: no one ever died of a chocolate deficiency.)

There are other foods you eat, though, that you might not be so emotional about. Eating a substitute instead of the real thing might be almost as satisfactory, and you'll save a lot of calories. For example:

● Tonic water adds 99 calories, bitter lemon 144 calories, and sweetened ginger ale adds 102 calories to mixed drinks. Mix all drinks with plain carbonated water, which has zero calories.

● Grape jam, when artificially sweetened, has about 4 calories per two tablespoons. Ordinary grape jam is up there at 35 calories for two tablespoons.

● Instead of eating fruit pie (around 410 calories a slice), bake an apple. Flavour it with cinnamon and low-cal raspberry fruit drink.

● Weight Watchers Fruit Cocktail has 50 calories per average serving. Compare that to Del Monte Fruit Cocktail at 170 calories per average serving.

● One normal chocolate cupcake has 101 calories per 1 oz/

25 g. Head for the fruit instead. 1 oz/25 g blackberries has 17 calories; 1 oz/25 g fresh apricots has 7 calories.

● Instead of using crackers or melba toast, slice raw courgette or cucumber into thin rounds as the base for hors d'oeuvres.

● Potatoes are good for you, but you can cut calories even more by eating turnips (or a combination of the two). 8 oz/225 g mashed turnips have 34.5 calories; mashed potatoes, 91. (No butter!)

● Whole milk is actually about 96–97 per cent fat free with only 3.25–3.7 per cent fat. Skim or low-fat milk has only 1–2 per cent fat.

● Skim milk has 89 calories per 8 fl oz/225 ml; low-fat milk about 102 calories; whole milk can vary in calorie count from between 150 to 161 calories per 8 fl oz/225 ml, depending on the fat content.

● Instead of whole milk and whole milk products, substitute: skim or low-fat milk, low-fat yogurt, buttermilk and polyunsaturated margarine (about ¾ tablespoon of oil equals 1 tablespoon of butter).

● Use low-calorie salad dressings.

● Soured cream substitute? It's possible. Blend one tablespoon of lemon juice and two tablespoons of skim milk into 8 oz/225 g low-fat cottage cheese.

● Feed the yolk of eggs to the dog or cat. (They're pretty much invulnerable to cholesterol problems.) Keep the white. Add two teaspoons of polyunsaturated oil to each egg white and beat. Use as a whole egg substitute.

● Flavour plain low-fat yogurt or low-fat cottage cheese with an eighth of a teaspoon of vanilla essence. It adds only 2½ calories.

21. Seasonal Guide to Dieter's Dilemmas

That word association test (on page 179) wasn't just for fun. We really do tend to associate names, places, events, and even problems with food. Christmas? It's a religious holiday, but it's also related to going home, seeing the family, and eating glazed ham, Christmas pudding and mince pies till you drop. New Year's Eve: as much as it's noisemakers, and teary reminiscence, it's also associated with caviar, vats of artillery punch, lobster salad, and an assortment of cheeses.

Let's keep going. Valentine's Day: chocolates, right? Easter? Roast spring lamb, simnel cake and chocolate Easter bunnies. June: you're in the mood for a picnic. It's warm, so you bring lots of sugary fruit drinks, potato crisps and easy-to-make sandwiches like tuna, heavy on the mayonnaise. July and August: you go to the beach and eat junk food or have a diet of junk food and ice creams. Harvest Festival means fancy breads and cakes and Hallowe'en provides an excuse for toffee apples and punch.

Somewhere in here was your birthday. What's a birthday without cake, ice cream and a few drinks?

Now, I wouldn't tell you to stop celebrating. You just have to stop making the association between holidays and food so that you are only looking forward to the goodies, not the day. You can start to see holidays as a time to *socialize* with good feelings rather than a time for feeling good from filling up.

How to be a diet-conscious guest in any season:

- When you go to a party or dinner, don't leave the house until you've eaten something first. That's right. Even if you're going out to a dinner, eat first. Have your snack.

Otherwise you may start allowing yourself to eat anything in sight with the excuse that you haven't eaten much – plus, if you've eaten, you won't be so hungry.

- If your hostess insists you sample her famous, homemade, calorie-laden whatever, decline graciously. If she further insists, ask her if there's a hospital in the vicinity. When she asks why, tell her you're allergic to the main ingredient and if you eat it, you'll die. It works every time.

- Your diet is your business. Don't tell anyone. Don't even whisper it. You don't want to start a conversation around the table about dieting. You will make yourself uncomfortable. (A few jokers will have a few unnecessary one-liners about fat.)

- If there is a dinner you especially want to go to *and* sample, cut back on calories at least a couple of days ahead of time. If you save up 300 or 400 calories on the cutback, you can have some of Aunt Gert's apple popover delight or a small wedge of Brie without trembling with guilt.

- If you want a drink, pour a *little* white wine into some salt-free soda and don't make yourself miserable by helping to prepare all these platters of food you can't touch. Instead, keep busy by arranging flowers, putting out the silver and glasses or keeping your hostess's kids amused and out of the way.

- Make socializing, and not the food, the focus of the party or dinner. That really is the point, after all.

Holiday Baking and Cooking

- Instead of giving baked goods as gifts, make decorations or things to wear.

- If you really enjoy holiday baking, give pies, breads and cakes rather than biscuits. Your friends will notice a cake with a piece missing, but may not be aware that their gift of 3 dozen iced biscuits started out from a recipe for 4 dozen.

- Make something you won't be tempted to snack on, like homemade chutney, relishes or mustard.

- When you mix cake batter and icing, don't scrape the bowl or pan for the remains. A rubber spatula is a great tool, but when it's got icing on it, it has a way of looking like a spoon. Don't lick it off.
- Tell your family it's time for a new (low-cal) holiday menu. No creamed anything. No brown-sugar anything. No glazes. No pies. No Grandma's old-fashioned butter shortbread.
- If your family wants to take you out for your birthday, splurge on filet mignon (5 oz/150 g, trimmed), one baked potato (no soured cream or butter), a green salad, and fresh melon for dessert. Toast with one glass of wine. Calories: under 500. No birthday cake – that can wait another year.

The author of *Jaws* **should know:** *Weight Watchers* magazine asked Peter Benchley how he avoided overeating under stress. Instead of heading for food, he told them, he puts on a pair of too-tight trousers that he keeps around. This gives him a 'first-hand account of what it feels like to grow out of one's clothes. It does the trick,' he said, 'I lose all desire to eat.'

22. Other Ways to Fry a Fish

There are better ways to do some of your old cooking chores – ways that help you get the most from food nutritionally and save the most calories. For example, a hint about cooking fish (I didn't really mean for you to fry it – I just thought the title would attract your attention) follows right now:

● If you rub a thinly sliced piece of fresh ginger over fish, you'll not only have a lovely ginger flavour, but less of a fish flavour.

● By now you know that if you refrigerate meat soups or stews, the fat solidifies. Since the fat's hardened on the surface, you can scoop it off. You can also skim off the fat while the stew's on the burner. Lower the flame a jot, then carefully put the pot half on and half off the burner. With cooler temperature on one side of the pot, the fat globules will have less chance to disperse throughout the stew. Result: the fat will accumulate on the cooler side. Be there with a spoon to skim it off.

● When you cook onions, turnips, beetroot, cabbage or greens, keep the lid off the pot. These vegetables don't like high heat. They react by giving off odours, and becoming slimy and overcooked.

● To preserve the vitamins in carrots when cooking them, cut them up, put them in a small pan with about ½ inch/1 cm water, cover, and simmer gently. They'll cook quicker, too. The aim is for them to soak up the water in which they were cooking so the nutrients aren't lost in cooking water that is discarded.

● Mashing potatoes and puréeing vegetables increases the loss of vitamin C – sometimes up to one-half of it is lost in the process. Cut them into chunks or eat them whole.

● Most of the vitamins in vegetables lie just under the skins. Don't pare them too deeply if you *do* pare them, or try to cook them with the skins.

● When you steam vegetables, let the water boil before you drop the veggies into the steamer. When steaming, allow an extra 3–5 minutes for cooking than when you use water to cover.

● Add butter to veggies when they're hot and toss immediately to distribute it evenly.

● Keep the water you've cooked veggies in and use for soups.

● Allow margarine to stand at room temperature before using it. Since it's softer, it can be spread thinner.

● When you grill meat (lean cuts only with the fat trimmed), don't salt it while it's under the heat. Salt draws out the natural juices.

● When spicing food with paprika or curry, watch the heat level. These spices scorch.

● Haul out your baking sheet from deep bun tins and pop whole stuffed green or red peppers into the cups. The hollows prevent the peppers from toppling over while cooking.

● Don't use bicarbonate of soda to preserve the natural colour of a vegetable. This just about ruins the nutritional value of the veggie, and adds sodium. Instead, if you're interested in aesthetics, add a drop of lemon juice, which should work just as well to preserve colour.

● Don't boil or overcook fruit – you're destroying the vitamin C. Boil water first, then drop fruit in. Turn the heat to low and simmer. Test the fruit so it's not at the mushy stage when it's cooked.

23. A Pat on Your (Thin) Back

They say that people like to eat when they are sad, depressed, or angry. If you're like me, you also celebrate with food. You give it to yourself as a reward when you're happy. Do these sound familiar?

I got a raise. (I'll have a couple of raised doughnuts.)
My trip to Spain is on. (I'll make a trip to the deli.)
My check-up was okay. (See you at the checkout counter.)

This kind of thinking is a no-no, unless you want to keep on gaining like a yo-yo. Stop right now. Reward yourself with anything but food. You'll be saving a lot of money by not eating the way you used to.

- Buy necessities, but make them the best – Givenchy pantyhose, A Dunhill toothbrush, hand-milled soap, a monogrammed washcloth or a small basket filled with potpourri for the bath.
- Buy a single place setting of china/crystal/flatware – the pattern that you've always wanted. As you reach different goal weights, add to the settings. If you have to lose a lot, here's the advantage: you'll end up with a full service of the most beautiful china, crystal, and flatware in town.
- Treat yourself to the best skin care products on the market.
- Hire a baby sitter for a few hours and browse around the best shops in town.
- If you do your own laundry, have everything sent out once in a while. What a luxury to have a closet full of neatly

ironed blouses you didn't have to slave over. Or ironed sheets for a change.

- Take a long lunch hour and go to a movie you're dying to see.
- Buy something you think is a real indulgence but one you've always wanted: an electric pencil sharpener, an embosser for your envelopes, personalized stationery.

24. A Note About Calorie Counters

I have used three major sources for calorie counts in this book: *Bowes and Church's Food Values of Portions Commonly Used* (Harper/Colophon), C. F. Adams' *Nutritive Value of American Foods* (Department of Agriculture, published November 1975), and Barbara Kraus' *Calories and Carbohydrates* (Signet). There are a lot of other calorie counters on the market – sometimes you can even get free ones from insurance companies – and I would say that most are pretty reliable.

Now don't be terribly concerned about the fact that your calorie counter and the caloric values that follow, or the ones you read in another book, don't always agree exactly. Each one may have minor variations, and for good reason. One is that produce grown (and tested) in different parts of the country may contain more or less simple sugar, depending on growing conditions, so the calorie count will differ. Also, the particular brand of food tested may differ: whole wheat bread tested by one laboratory may contain different ingredients or ingredients in different proportions than the whole wheat bread tested by another.

The food exchange programme on pages 128-9 is designed to help you select foods without having to think about the calories, but I know that some of you would like to have a handy reference for caloric values of common foods. So here goes:

BRIEF CALORIE COUNTER

Apple, 1 medium (2½ inch/6 cm diameter)	80
Apple sauce, unsweetened, 4 fl oz/120 ml	50

Artichokes, Jerusalem, 2½ oz/70 g, sliced	10
Asparagus, 1 spear	4
Aubergine, 2 oz/50 g	15
Bacon rashers, back, grilled, 1 oz/25 g	101
streaky, grilled, 1 oz/25 g	106
Banana, medium (6 inch/15 cm)	90
Beans, green, 1½ oz/40 g	25
Beef, sirloin or hamburger, lean, 1 oz/25 g	
after cooking	60
Beetroot, about 3½ oz/85 g	15
Bread, whole wheat, 1 thin slice	40
Broccoli, 4 spears	40
Brussels sprouts, 4	20
Butter, 1 T.	100
Cabbage, raw, 3 oz/ 75 g	15
Cantaloupe, ¼	35
Carrot, 1 medium whole	20
Cauliflower, 2½ oz/70 g	10
Celery, 1 large outer stalk or 3 small inner	10
Cereal	
Bran flakes, ¾ oz/20 g	75
Rice Krispies, ¾ oz/20 g	75
Rolled oats, 1 oz/25 g	100
Puffed Rice, ¾ oz/20 g	75
Puffed Wheat, ¾ oz/20 g	75
Cherries, 4 oz/100 g	40
Cheese, Parmesan, 1 T.	30
Chicken, 1 oz/25 g skinned and boned breast, raw	50
Clams, 1 oz/25 g	25
Cod or mullet, raw, 7 oz/200 g	190
Cottage cheese, low-fat, 4 oz/113 g	100
Courgette, 6 oz/175 g	20
Crabmeat, 1 oz/25 g	30
Cranberries, 2 oz/50 g	25
Cucumber, ½	10
Egg, whole	75
Egg, white only	15

Flounder, 1 oz/25 g	25
Grapefruit, ½	40
Green beans, 2½ oz/70 g	15
Green pepper, 1 large	20
Hamburger, lean, raw, 1 oz/ 25 g after grilling	60
Honeydew melon, ½	60
Lamb, 5 oz/150 g chop after grilling	125
Lemon, 1 medium	30
Lettuce, ½ head	20
Liver, beef or calf, 1 oz/25 g	40
Liver, chicken, 1 oz/25 g	50
Lime, 1 medium	30
Lobster, 1 oz/25 g	30
Margarine, 1 T.	100
Mayonnaise, low-calorie, 1 T.	40
Mayonnaise, regular, 1 T.	100
Melba toast, 1 slice	15
Milk, skim, 8 fl oz/225 ml	90
Mushrooms, 4 oz/100 g	30
Mustard, 1 T.	15
Nectarine, 1 medium	35
Noodles, egg, 3 oz/75 g	200
Oatmeal, cooked, 6 oz/175 g	100
Okra, 3 oz/75 g	50
Olives, green, medium, 2	15
Olive, ripe, large, 1	20
Onion, raw, 1 oz/25 g	15
Onion, raw, 1 T.	5
Onion, boiled, 2 oz/50 g	30
Orange, 1 medium	80
Orange juice concentrate, 2 tsp.	10
Oysters, 1 oz/25 g	20
Pear, 1 medium	120
Peach, 1 medium	40
Pepper, green, large, 1	20
Pineapple, canned, packed in water, 1 slice	40
Pineapple, packed in unsweetened juice, 1 slice	60

Plum, 1 medium, blue	50
Pork, 1 oz/25 g after grilling	60
Popcorn (no oil), ½ oz/15 g	55
(with 4 T. oil), ½ oz/15 g	80
Potato, 1 medium (approx. 5½ oz/160 g)	90
Prawns, canned, 7 oz/198 g	230
Raisins, 1 T.	30
Rhubarb, fresh, unsweetened, 5 oz/150 g	10
Rice, cooked, 8 oz/225 g	160
Salmon, 1 oz/25 g	60
Scallops, raw, 6 oz/175 g	190
Shrimp, raw, 1 oz/25 g	25
Sole, 1 oz/25 g	25
Spinach, boiled, 3½ oz/85 g	20
Spring onion, 1 small	4
Steak, 1 oz/25 g	60
Strawberries, 4 oz/100 g	50
Tangerine, 1 medium	40
Tomato, fresh, 1 medium	30
Trout, 1 oz/25 g	50
Tuna, in brine, 6½ oz/186 g	220
Turkey, 1 oz/25 g	50
Veal, 1 oz/25 g	100
Watermelon, 1 6×1-inch/15×2.5-cm slice	100
Yogurt, plain, 4 oz/100 g	70
Yogurt, vanilla, 4 oz/100 g	100

*NOTE: Except where indicated, weights for meat and fish are for cooked portions weighed without bone, skin, shell or fat; meat should be lean and trimmed and skin of poultry should be removed before cooking.

DIET DIARY

Today is _____

I've been helping myself for _____ days

EATING

Time of Day	Food	Calories
Breakfast (a.m.)		
Lunch ( )		
Dinner ( )		
Fourth Meal ( )		

TOTAL CALORIES: _____

Notes on today:

Goals for tomorrow:

WALKING

Time of Day	Warm-up (Mins.)	Walking (Mins.)	Pulse Rate During Aerobic Walk	Distance Covered	Calories Burned

TOTAL CALORIES BURNED BY WALKING: _____

A Final Thought

You have probably heard of Pavlov's famous experiment. The Russian scientist rang a bell every time he was about to feed his laboratory dogs. Eventually, they came to connect the sound of the bell with the expectation of food, and the ringing of the bell alone was enough to start them salivating. Pavlov called this a conditioned reflex.

That's how some of us respond to the problem of being fat – by conditioned reflex rather than rational thought.

But consider this: Pavlov carried his experiment a step further. He taught his dogs to unlearn their response. He rang bells and *didn't* bring dinner and after a while that sound became a neutral one.

Stop being ruled by the bells.

Index

Index

Index